Healing Your Life:
Lessons on the Path of Ayurveda

By Dr. Marc Halpern

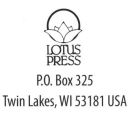

P.O. Box 325
Twin Lakes, WI 53181 USA

DISCLAIMER

This book is not intended to treat, diagnose or prescribe. The information contained herein is in no way to be considered as a substitute for a consultation with a duly licensed health care professional.

ALL RIGHTS RESERVED. No part of this book may be reproduced in any form or by any electronic or mechanical means including information storage and retrieval systems without permission in writing from the publisher, except by a reviewer who may quote brief passages in a review.

Author: Dr. Marc Halpern

Copyright © 2011

First Edition 2011
Printed in the United States of America
ISBN: 978-0-9102-6198-2
Library Of Congress Number: 2010926700

Published by:

Lotus Press, P.O. Box 325, Twin Lakes, WI 53181 USA
web: www.lotuspress.com
Email: lotuspress@lotuspress.com
800.824.6396

CONTENTS

FOREWORD

I have spent the last 25 years healing my life. Aside from any other qualifications I may have to write this book, that may be the most important. Along the way, my journey has led to healers of many traditions, countless books and a variety of personal growth workshops. My journey also took me into the heart of professional healing itself as I became a Chiropractor and then participated in post-graduate studies of Chinese Medicine, Homeopathy, Herbalism and Ayurvedic Medicine. Beyond my professional journey, my journey to heal myself lead me to additional bodies of healing knowledge including psychic healing, tai chi, and holotropic breath work. My thirst for knowledge was not quenched, however, and I continued down a road that eventually brought me to Ayurveda and yoga. Having drunk from that well, I have tasted water that is both sweet and divinely nourishing. My journey today is taking me deeper and deeper down that well.

Like churning cream into butter and clarifying butter into ghee, my body, mind and consciousness has undergone transformation after transformation to get to where it is today. Today, I am happier, healthier and I experience a degree of inner peace that I never suspected was possible. This book is in many ways a summary of the most important knowledge I have gained on my journey. While the introduction tells of my personal healing journey, this book is not meant to be a complete memoir. It is only a glimpse into the world I have walked and the lessons I have learned.

This book is a road map. If you follow it, it will lead you toward optimal health and greater peace of mind. If that is what you want, you have picked up the right book. This book does not provide shortcuts, only clarity. As you read this book, please remember that I am not the one who has created this road map. I am not the originator of this knowledge. This map has been around for thousands of years. All I have done is present it to you with as much clarity as I can. I, too, am a traveler along its path.

This book is first and foremost dedicated to the ancient rishis (teachers) of India who shared what they learned about optimal health and peace of mind with their students. And, to their students who became teachers and passed this knowledge and wisdom on to the next generation. And so on and so on through the ages so that this knowledge is available today. I would like to thank all of the teachers who have personally inspired me on this journey, including Swami Sivananda of Rishikesh, whose writings and legacy unlocked many doors in my consciousness. Vamadeva Shastri (Dr. David Frawley), who christened my ship as I set sail on my ayurvedic journey in 1992, established the foundation of my training and has always supported my work. Swami Vishnu Devananda, founder of the Sivananda Yoga Vedanta Society, from whose heart a lotus has sprung with petals unfolding around the world. And, Dr. Subhash Ranadé whose time spent with me in my home helped clarify many pieces of ayurvedic knowledge.

I would also like to thank each teacher who over the years has come to the California College of Ayurveda and deposited a piece of their knowledge and experience, including: Dr. Avinash Lélé, Dr. Akhilesh Sharma, Dr. Liladhar Gupta, Dr. Vasant Lad, Dr. John Douillard, Dr. Frank Ros, Kim McCarthy and Kathi Keville.

I wish to thank my students for trusting me and for coming to the California College of Ayurveda to study. Since 1995, when the College opened its doors, you have provided me with a field and forum to play with and explore this knowledge. Your questions over more than a decade have inspired me to go deeper and deeper into the well of truth and knowledge.

Most of all, I would like to thank my family: My two children, Jordy and Bryce, from whom I have learned the true meaning of unconditional love. And, my wife Kristin, who has nurtured and supported me and without whom I might not be alive today.

PREFACE

The current health and ecological crisis in our global society is likely to increase in the years to come as the population grows and as unhealthy urban lifestyles proliferate throughout the world. Perhaps the best solution for this growing problem can be found in a return to traditional natural healing systems and readjusting our lives according to them, restoring once more our balance with the world of nature.

One of the most significant of all such natural healing systems is Ayurveda, the traditional medicine of India. Ayurveda has an experiential history of over five thousand years as an integral part of the civilization of India and South Asia. It is recognized as one of the world's main medical system by the World Health Organization (WHO) and remains widely practiced in India today. Over the past few decades Ayurveda has spread worldwide and now Ayurvedic centers can be found in most major cities and countries of the world.

Ayurveda's appeal is closely connected with Yoga, which millions of people worldwide are taking up for its health benefits. In fact, Ayurveda is the traditional yogic system of medicine. It is based upon the same philosophy and principles as Yoga but has developed these into a full system of preventative and curative medicine.

Ayurveda is very different from and covers much more of our lives than medicine as we ordinarily conceive it to be. Ayurveda is first of all a science of right living and only secondarily a system for treating acute diseases. Ayurveda teaches us the principles of harmonious living in balance with nature, society, our own individual constitution and the universal consciousness. Ayurveda does not begin with the treatment of disease but rather with an examination of life patterns and our role in the cosmic web of existence. Based on that deeper vision, Ayurveda does address how to treat specific diseases but from a foundation of oneness and wholeness with all that takes us beyond the strategy of conflict and confrontation that much of medicine has adopted in its effort to fight disease. The Ayurvedic practitioner or doctor is a life-counselor who can guide us to optimal well-being for all aspects of our life, not simply a specialist who can treat one disease or another.

In this book, Dr. Marc Halpern takes a broad view of Ayurveda and shows us how to apply it in the context of modern life. Dr. Halpern is one of America's most important pioneers of Ayurvedic education. He established the California College of Ayurveda in 1995, which was the first institution in the United States to go beyond teaching Ayurveda for self-healing and teach the clinical aspects of Ayurveda to its students. His school developed the first Clinical Ayurvedic Specialist title recognized by the state of California that has become a model for other Ayurvedic schools in North America and in Europe.

Starting schools, particularly in such a new subject, is not an easy task. Yet Dr. Halpern has persisted and been successful. He has developed important curriculums for Ayurvedic training as well as special text books for advanced study. He has helped develop the main associations involved in promoting Ayurveda like the National Association of Ayurvedic Medicine (NAMA) and the California Association of Ayurvedic Medicine (CAAM).

I have known Marc since 1992, when he first came to me as a student seeking deeper knowledge in Ayurveda. He trained and worked with me for several years and I have remained in touch with him on a regular basis and serve as an advisor for his school. I have observed Marc over the years and seen his determination and dedication in the cause of Ayurveda.

Marc's current book Healing Your Life strives to make Ayurveda understandable to a broader audience, not just as a means of treating disease but as a means of gaining mastery over our entire lives. He communicates the insights and healing tools that he has gained in his many years teaching and practicing Ayurveda. The book is divided into lessons, not simply chapters, which represent the author's distillation of the wisdom of Ayurveda in its practical application that any discerning reader can apply with great benefits.

The book is particularly relevant to the lifestyle aspect of Ayurveda, which is the first and primary level on which Ayurveda must be applied in order to really work. Ayurveda begins with the principles of healthy, natural, happy, creative and spiritual living, which if we follow will reduce, if not eliminate, most of the ailments that are likely to befall us through the course of our lives. The reader may be surprised at the scope of the Ayurvedic view of health and well-being that covers such diverse topics as the proper use of the senses and special sensory therapies, like color therapy, which modern medicine rarely considers. Marc addresses this Ayurvedic approach to the senses in detail, probably more so than in any other of the available books on Ayurveda. According to Ayurveda, the misuse of the senses is one of the main causes of disease and their proper use one of the most important aspects of treatment.

Healing Your Life covers a notable range of topics from diet to psychology with clarity, detail and adaptability. It shows a living Ayurveda connected to our daily experience, a system of medicine that we can live and grow with throughout our lives, not something imposed upon us from the outside against our natural functioning. The book is as much a personal journey as it is a teaching manual. Healing Your Life serves as an excellent introduction to Marc's work as well as to the field of Ayurveda as a whole. It can help you gain mastery of your own happiness and well-being, which is your real birthright.

Dr. David Frawley
Author: *Yoga and Ayurveda, Ayurvedic Healing*

Introduction:

Healing My Life: A Personal
Journey into the Cause of Disease

Healing the world begins with healing yourself

Who knows what road they will walk, where they will go and how they will get there? I'm 47 years old and I had no idea that during my life I'd travel to Hell and back again; a journey from tremendous pain and suffering to remarkable well-being. But then this journey is not over. There is no choice but to walk forward.

In many ways, my journey began when I was about 12 years old. At least, this is when I became a conscious participant in it. My father asked me what I wanted to be when I grew up. He had asked me this question before and previously, I had always answered him with something fanciful, such as being a baseball player. After all, I grew up in New York, was a fan of the New York Yankees and my hero was Mickey Mantle. I remember well his last game. I was there. This time, however, after a moment of reflection, I looked him in the eye and said, "Dad, what I really want to be is happy." From that moment onward, being happy became the main criteria for how I would choose my career.

Looking back, I realize that I answered his question the way I did because all around me I saw people who appeared to be unhappy and unhealthy. Some might say that complaining is just a part of a normal New York Jewish upbringing. It's a tradition. But it wasn't just my family that seemed unhappy. I was aware that the world around me was suffering. Through the newspapers and television I saw the end of the Vietnam war and the assassinations of Martin Luther King (on my birthday) and Robert Kennedy. I also observed the mundane hour-long commute my father would take each day as he drove from upstate New York to the Bronx as a high school social studies teacher. My parents were not happy in their relationship either. To say the least, I was less than inspired to grow up and be a part of that world.

I decided then that I would keep my eyes open for something I could do when I grew up that would contribute to making me happy and perhaps contribute to helping others along the way. Of course, I had no idea at the time that so much of the suffering I perceived in others was a reflection of the suffering I was experiencing deep inside myself. I had no idea that there was no job that could make a person happy. And, I certainly had no idea that my journey to understand how to end the suffering was going to be a journey that would first bring all of my own suffering to the surface to face and fully experience. I had no idea that this was part of the process of healing.

How many teachers does one person need? Some say only one and when you meet your teacher you must surrender completely. I've never met the One, but I've had many teachers along the way. Some have taught information and increased my knowledge of the ordinary physical world. Others have taught me "life lessons" such as integrity through their way of being. Their impact was deeper helping to shape my personality. And then there are those most special teachers who have helped me to understand the mysteries that lie beyond the reach of the ordinary senses. They've helped me to expand my idea of who I am and my relationship to the world around me. Sometimes those teachers have helped facilitate extraordinary experiences. Others have helped me to understand the extraordinary experiences that found me. My life has been filled with extraordinary experiences and some of them quite mystical. Whether as a child perceiving my own subtle energy body, as a pre-teen experiencing dramatic and long lasting déjà-vu or as a teenager or as young adult opening the doors of perception with psychedelic drugs, the extraordinary always seemed to find me and, at the time, seemed rather ordinary.

Teachers began to show up in my life when I was about 12 years old to help me explain some of the extraordinary experiences I was having. I didn't recognize them as teachers at the time, just interesting people with interesting ideas. One of the more important teachers was Ernie Landie, a New York Chiropractor. I went to see him after struggling with shoulder and neck pain that was interfering with my ability to play high school baseball. He was different from anyone I'd ever met. To me, he seemed happy, healthy and excited about life. And, most of all, he was excited about Chiropractic and its ability to bring health and well-being to others. He believed that if everyone got a chiropractic adjustment and removed the neurological interference between the brain and the body that the world would be a happier and healthier place.

After noting my interest, he invited me to go with him on a trip from New York to South Carolina for a week to visit Sherman Chiropractic College where I spent a week with some of the great minds in the field of Chiropractic. I listened to lectures that inspired me in ways I had never been inspired before. From these great teachers I learned my first model for understanding the cause of suffering. I learned that disease was caused by a separation between man-the-physical and man-the-spiritual – a separation between universal intelligence and personal or innate intelligence. And, I learned that the way to correct this separation was through the Chiropractic adjustment. If this does not seem like typical Chiropractic to you, you are not alone; I later found out that I was spending time with a small but very special group of chiropractors.

I began my formal studies in Chiropractic at the age of 21. In 1983, after spending three years at the University of Buffalo in New York where I studied the basic sciences, I got into my green Pontiac Tempest and began a month long, National Park filled journey across the country enroot to California to attend Palmer College of Chiropractic-West. Among my first classes was a class in philosophy. While I enjoyed the class, to my surprise, half the students in class protested that these traditional philosophical principles of healing were being taught at all. They felt there was no place in the "science" of Chiropractic for this quasi-spiritual philosophy. And they were not alone. I found out that much of the profession felt similarly. That class was the last I heard of these principles till much later. And so, I immersed myself in the world of science and found great joy in learning the details of how the body functioned.

Three years later, at the age of 24, I began my internship at the College's clinic. As I walked into the treatment room for the first time, it struck me: I didn't know what I was doing. I knew how to adjust the spine. I knew how to make pops and clicks in the vertebra. What I didn't know was how this was going to really help people to become happier and healthier. I could analyze the spine and figure out what vertebrae needed to be adjusted but I had forgotten the teachings of that small group of chiropractors I had met at the age of 16. I became depressed and when I'm depressed I go to the mountains.

I took an early morning hike in a nearby mountain range called Rancho San Antonio State Park. The highest peak was not very high but it overlooked the Bay Area south of San Francisco. I decided that I would sit there and, for the first time in my life, I would pray to God. I was not at all religious but I decided that I needed some spiritual guidance. I was depressed, and when we become depressed, sometimes we find ourselves open to Divine intervention. This was one of those times. I had no idea what would take place. I did not know if I would see a burning bush, an old man with a beard, or if perhaps a coyote would come out of the forest and speak to me. I was open to whatever would happen. I decided I would sit quietly and hold the question I had out to God, who I hoped would appear in some form and give me an answer. The question I had was this: "What do I need to know about healing right now?" I had no idea how long that would take. I sat for several hours and soon the noon hour passed and there was no sign of God. I sat for several more hours and still there was no sign of God. The dinner hour passed and the sun was starting to set. My patience exhausted, I became even more depressed, as it seemed that God had forsaken me. I was not prepared to stay overnight and so I stood up, let go of my question, and began my slow descent down the switch backs of the mountain.

I will never forget the moment I turned one particular switch back. I stopped suddenly as I heard a voice. The voice was as clear as if someone were standing next to me speaking. I quickly realized that, although the voice appeared to be separate from me, it was speaking to me from within. The voice gave me a clear answer. This was profound to me for two reasons. One was the answer I received. The more profound reason, however, was that this was my first direct perception of the Divine beginning a relationship that would become deeper and deeper over time. From that moment on, I began to look to the Divine for guidance.

The answer that I received was a simple one. I needed to learn to unconditionally love each patient who came to see me. And that if I did, my hands would be guided to where they needed to be and something extra would flow through me from above down and from the inside out when I touched them, and this "something" would bring healing to them. In that moment, my heart opened and somewhat like the proverbial Grinch, it grew several sizes bigger that day. I walked back to my car with a spring in my step. I went back to the clinic and knew that my patients would get well. And they did. But my learning was only just beginning.

Just before graduation, I came down with a mysterious illness that quickly left me crippled with severe joint pain throughout my body. One morning, I woke up with pain in my left ankle. I could not remember injuring it. That day, I limped my way through school. The next day, the pain was completely gone but my other ankle hurt so much that again I had to limp. I had studied enough medicine to know that pain was not supposed to shift from one part of one's body to the other and I became greatly concerned. Sometimes, even those of us who are more alternatively minded, when faced with a potentially serious illness reflexively and urgently feel that we need to see a "real" doctor. This was one of those times. So, I went to the only one I knew, a physician who worked at our school. After I told him my symptoms, I recall his thoughts very well. They were profound to me for all the wrong reasons. "Well Marc," he said. "Statistically, young men of your age with migrating arthritis have a condition called Gonococcal Arthritis, a form of Gonorrhea. All you need is a shot of penicillin and you will be well." This was profound to me first and foremost because I was a "statistic". I was also baffled by the diagnosis, as I was not sexually active outside of the relationship I was in. And I was as sure as I could be that my girlfriend was not either. Even so, I went to his office for a shot. On the way out of his office, I passed out. My body experienced an anaphylactic reaction to the antibiotic. Anaphylaxis is a severe and potentially life-threatening allergic reaction that causes one's blood pressure to rapidly drop. After a shot of epinephrine, I awoke in the doctor's office with a rash from head to toe. He assured me that I would be all right and that the medicine would still work. So, I went home.

Each day, my symptoms became worse. The pain moved to my knees and then to my elbows and wrists and eventually began affecting two joints, and then three joints, until eventually it affected virtually my entire body.

I began to rapidly lose weight, my liver stopped working properly and I became anemic. I also developed allergies to the world around me, including the sun itself. Within a few weeks, I was left bedridden, unable to walk and in the greatest pain of my life. In the morning my body was stiff like a board. By the afternoon the real pain would set in and even a bed sheet on my body would cause excruciating pain. I saw specialists in rheumatology and immunology at Stanford University who, while being able to measure the dysfunctions in my blood, were unable to determine any cause for what was happening. I appeared at the Grand Rounds where a group of physicians come together and discuss the odd and unusual and try to figure out what is going on. It was apparent that no one knew why I was sick, and that there were no ideas for how to bring about healing. A recommendation was made that I should be hospitalized and given drugs that would suppress my immune system in an attempt to control the inflammation. There was a risk of serious side effects from the treatment. I was at a crossroad.

Several days earlier in bed in my apartment, I began mourning the loss of the life that I thought I was going to live. I began letting go of the idea that I would have a successful practice, get married and have kids. I began to resign myself to either being crippled the rest of my life or perhaps dying. I began to cry. As the tears flowed, I heard a voice speak to me. I recognized it immediately as the voice I had heard walking on the trails of the mountain nearly a year before. "Everything will be OK," it said. "You will have to go on a journey to learn how to heal yourself. For you, all of the diplomas on the wall will not matter. When you learn how to heal yourself, only then you will know how to heal others." In a sense, this was a final examination given to me by God. Pass and I get to move on and help others. Fail and I, well, die. For some reason, in that moment, that seemed OK too.

I had to make a decision. Go into the hospital and surrender to the medical treatments or begin the journey to heal myself. I chose the road less traveled and that was the last time that I saw a physician for my illness.

My journey led me many places. I explored the major forms of alternative healing, such as Chiropractic, Acupuncture, and Homeopathy, but they did not help me. I even tried fasting for ten days on beet, carrot and celery juice. This did not help either and I only lost more weight. Then, a friend of mine said I should see someone he knew, a psychic healer by the name of Greg Schelkun in San Rafael, California. I was not a great believer in psychic healing but I had nothing to lose. So, my girlfriend, whom I was living with at the time, drove me to see him.

My visit was short, perhaps only 15 minutes and he lightly touched different parts of my body. Then he said he was done and he helped me to sit up. Seeing as how he was supposed to be "psychic", I asked him what he did, what was wrong with me and what I could expect to happen next. His answer surprised me. I had expected a rather generalized, perhaps cryptic response that I would have to find meaning in -- the type of response that could apply to many people. Instead he told me this. He said that it was as if my body's immune system had a dead battery and he gave it a jump start. "Tonight," he said, "your body temperature will rise up to 105 and you will have tremendous night sweats, and then in the morning you will be fine." I was rather surprised that he made such a specific prediction. I wasn't sure what to say after that. He told me that this was the first of three great challenges that I would have in my life. He didn't tell me what the others would be.

I went home and that night I put a towel between me and the bed just in case I really did experience great night sweats. I awoke in the middle of the night and the towel was dry. I awoke the next morning and still the towel was dry. I had no great fever (I had been running a consistent 99 degrees) and did not have night sweats. I called up Greg and told him that nothing had happened. He said that I needed another jump start. I explained to him that I could not travel again (it took all of my energy to get to his office) and so he told me to just sit still and that he would heal me from where he was. I thought that this was getting stranger and stranger. After rolling my eyes, I did as he said. I sat quietly in meditation and I was surprised to feel heat in my body where he had touched me the previous day. I thought that maybe it was my imagination remembering the heat from his hands. That night I went to bed and placed another towel between my body and the bed. Sure enough, in the middle of the night, my fever rose and I had great night sweats. Greg was almost right.

My fever rose to 105 degrees but it did not come down. My fever fluctuated between 103.5 and 105.5 for the next two weeks and now I appeared at times somewhat catatonic as well as crippled. I took fluids but barely ate. I lay in bed all day hardly able to move or talk. Then, something happened.

What I experienced next is hard to explain. I lay there in bed and found myself observing myself. It was as if some part of me was separated from the rest of me. No, I was not hovering like a ghost, though that comes to mind and others might describe the experience in that way. I found myself distant and separated from my body. I was examining myself and saying, "Look at you, look at what a mess you are. All you ever wanted was to be happy and healthy and now look at you." At that moment, it dawned on me that the part of me that was observing me, the observer, was perfect and unaffected by the illness.

I continued to look at myself through those eyes. As I observed my body, I realized that it was no longer solid. My body appeared as a dense field of energy. Within that field, there was a flow to the energy. As I observed it more closely I noticed that in each area of pain there were blockages to the flow of energy. There were also blockages to the flow in my liver and spleen. All I could do at first was be a witness to these observations. Over time however, I realized that the part of me that appeared separate from what was going on could also interact with and ultimately control that field of energy. Through what I can best describe as a combination of awareness and intention, I learned that I could affect the flow of energy in my body and undo the blockages. Once I learned that, I turned an important corner.

I spent most of each day observing the flow of the energy through my body. I removed the blockages to the flow of energy and repeated it each time the flow became obstructed again. Each time, the channels of flow remained un-blocked for a longer and longer period of time. As energy flowed into the tissues of my body that were suffering, I felt them become more alive and I felt them beginning to heal themselves. After a couple of weeks, my body temperature came down, my pain lessened and I worked my way into a wheelchair and then back to walking and moving about the world once again.

I was very sick when I graduated from school in June of 1987 but I was mostly well by the time I took my State Board Exams in January and went to work in the field of Chiropractic. Even then though, I was not completely well. I was over the acute part of my condition but I was exhausted. I suffered from what most people now call Chronic Fatigue Syndrome. For the next seven years, from 1988 to 1995, I had to take afternoon naps, my body was very sensitive to the environment, I experienced frequent, though relatively mild reoccurrences of pain and my eyes often appeared half closed and red. For a few hours each morning and a few hours each afternoon though, I began to practice Chiropractic.

Through the experience of my illness and some additional guidance I received from another mentor, Dr. Robert Linford, I expanded on my ability to perceive and work with the flow of energy in my own body and learned how to work with the flow of energy in other people's bodies. I began to integrate this ability into the chiropractic work I was doing as I was now quite confident that I understood the cause of suffering and disease and that I had a methodology to remove it. I came to understand that disease was caused by blockages to the flow of energy in the body (through the nervous system and the subtle energy body) and that the purpose of my work was to help restore the natural flow of energy in the body. I did this through the chiropractic adjustment and through the laying on of hands.

Almost all of the patients that I treated got well and many of them made remarkable recoveries from both acute and chronic diseases. I saw one patient heal simultaneously from both Parkinson's disease and cancer. It was obvious that I was not the healer. It was apparent that when the flow of energy was normalized, the human body healed itself and I was honored to play a supporting role in the process.

My practice in Burlingame, California, just south of San Francisco, grew rapidly and I became very successful in a short period of time. I was busy seeing about 150 patients every week. Many came in for what I called maintenance and I gave them a tune up and made sure that the energy was flowing well in their bodies. Then, one patient suffered a heart attack between visits. I became confused, wondering how this happened. How could a person have a heart attack if their energy was flowing well through their heart!? Then it dawned on me. My patients have to keep coming back to me to restore the natural flow of energy. Something is happening when they leave my office that once again blocks up the flow of energy. I realized then that I was not treating the cause of disease and suffering. I realized that blocked energy is a symptom of something else. This was very disturbing to me. My path was not to treat the symptom but to remove the cause. Once again, I became depressed and went to the mountains.

It was 1990 and I was twenty-eight years old. I went camping and hiking in Big Sur, California. While carrying a backpack on my back and firewood in my arms, I severely herniated two disks in my lower back and could not stand upright. Through a combination of crawling, laying down for rests and being carried, I made it back to my car. The same girlfriend who took care of me when I was crippled the first time, and who was now my wife drove me back to San Mateo, where we lived at the time. I spent the next three months in bed, unable to stand at times for more than 10 or 15 seconds. Although surgery was an option, my Chiropractic training had taught me that surgery was a road that once you drive down, you can never go back. It is a road that rarely leads to complete recovery and often causes serious complications. I decided to try and heal myself by allowing energy to flow into the disk without obstruction. After three months of bed rest, visits from my Chiropractor friends and deep meditation to keep the flow of energy around my disk free of obstruction, I was again on my feet and returned to my practice. My first patient was a large woman; when I bent over to adjust her hips, I re-injured my back and found myself in bed for yet another month. This became my story for most of the following year. I worked a month and then I was in bed a month. I am truly not sure which was worse, being crippled with the arthritic condition in my body or being crippled by the low back pain. I knew one thing through, that I was neither happy nor healthy. In fact, I was miserable.

One Friday, I drove to work in my little sports car and took my eye off of the narrow canyon road just long enough for a gust of wind to blow my car to the side of the road. My car climbed the bank and then rolled over several times before coming to rest on the roof. My windows shattered, I found myself upside down suspended by my safety belt. After realizing I was mostly ok, I looked for a way out and climbed through the shattered back window to the side of the road where I lay down and waited for help to arrive.

I was taken to the hospital and, thankfully, I was fine. I went home, rested and returned to work on Monday. That is when an angel in the form of a woman named Cindy knocked on my door. Cindy was a massage therapist, healer and clairvoyant psychic. She worked with me in my office and often worked on me as well. Cindy stuck her head into my office and, in her gentle manner said, "Excuse me, Dr. Halpern, it's none of my business, but would you like to know what is going on?" I told her to come in and she sat down and began to tell me the story of my life. She explained that there was more for me to do and that until I got on my path I would continue to suffer. She wasn't sure what I was supposed to do but said that running a chiropractic practice was not it and that it seemed to her to be much larger. Anyway, she said, until you are on your proper path, you will suffer. This is how the Divine is guiding you.

I told her that I knew that I was to do something different and that I wanted to find and remove the cause of disease and suffering. I also told her that I needed money and that in about five years I would be financially able to give up the practice and start on that journey. She listened and simply said, "Well, I just wanted you to know." And she left. I went on practicing and suffering working a month and then laying down for a month. I still suffered from Chronic Fatigue as well. I soon realized that I had no choice. I needed to sell the practice, so I could heal myself.

Surprisingly, no one came along to buy my practice. It was a beautiful office and a thriving practice in the San Francisco Bay Area and it should have sold quickly. Yet, no one seemed very interested. One day, Cindy knocked on my door and peeked inside. With her gentle heart she said, "Excuse me, Dr. Halpern, it's none of my business, but would you like to know why your practice won't sell?" "Come in" I said. Cindy told me that, until I let go of the practice in my heart, there would be no space for anyone else to buy it. I asked her, "Do you mean that, because I think that it wouldn't be so bad if my practice doesn't sell - because then in about 5 years I'll be financially independent and out of debt..... . She gently interrupted and said, "I just wanted to let you know" and she left.

That night I thought about what she said and decided that I really did want to sell my practice, end the day-to-day suffering and begin my journey toward my own health and whatever was next. I sat in meditation that night and imagined a cord from my heart to my practice and, in my mind, I cut that cord. When I did, I let go of my attachment to the practice. I also decided that I would close my doors and move on whether I sold my practice or not. I would tell my staff the next day at lunch.

I went into the office that next morning lighter and clearer, having already removed the burden of my practice from my consciousness. The phone rang shortly after I arrived. A woman on the other end said, "I heard your practice is for sale. If it is all that I've heard, I am very interested. I want to come by at lunch and see it today. Would that be ok?" Of course I said yes. "Oh and how soon do you want to be out of the practice?" she asked. Casually I responded, "Oh, whenever it seems right. When do you want to be in practice?" "Right away" she stated. My heart leaped in both fear and joy. I cancelled my lunch meeting with my staff and she came by at noon. Two weeks later, I was out of a job, floating within the void of empty space. What next?

I sat in meditation and prayed each evening. My prayer was a simple one. I prayed that my path would unfold before me and that I would have the courage to walk it. I was smart enough to know that these were two different things. Too often the path unfolds but the courage is lacking. And too often the courage is there but we are too blind to see the signs. I prayed for both. I also looked up toward God and said, "That's it, I surrender. All I ever wanted was to be happy and healthy and I am neither. I have a bad back, Chronic Fatigue and a fragile immune system. When I drive, all I seem to do is crash.

I give up. I want you to drive. I want to be in the back seat. Show me the path and give me the courage to walk it and I will serve. I know it won't always be easy and I won't complain. I surrender." I didn't realize it at the time, but, in that moment in 1991, I turned my life over to God.

A few days later, a flyer came in the mail for a six month post-graduate program being offered through New York College of Chiropractic, where I could learn the tenets of Homeopathy, Chinese medicine, Herbalism and something I had never heard of before: Ayurveda. I thought this was a good sign and that perhaps I could discover the true cause of disease from these disciplines. I engaged in the study of each discipline and it was when I began to study Ayurveda that something very special happened.

It was as if I began to remember everything I ever knew. Ayurveda unlocked the door to my heart and out flowed knowledge long forgotten from my childhood and perhaps from places long before that. Ayurveda gave language to what I already knew to be true and helped me remember what I had forgotten. Something told me I was on the right track and would eventually understand the cause of disease and suffering.

After completing that program, I sought out a teacher in Ayurveda and so I contacted Dr. David Frawley, the director of the American Institute of Vedic Studies. Out of work and supported by disability benefits, I was able to spend the next few years engaged in the full time study of Ayurveda. Ayurveda became an obsession. It was all I thought about and all I read about. I completed Dr. Frawley's correspondence course, read every book published in the United States on the subject, and probed him for answers to the endless questions that I had. I then participated in a residential week-long seminar he held in Santa Fe, New Mexico, where he had invited several ayurvedic doctors from India and other teachers of Ayurveda. Motivated by an inner realization that I was flowing on a path guided by something greater than myself, I pursued knowledge like a fire in pursuit of new fuel to burn.

I began to apply the principles of Ayurveda to my own healing process. I began to heal on the deepest of levels. I also began to attend yoga classes in San Francisco with a wonderful yoga teacher named Donna Farhi. Through these classes, my daily ayurvedic practices, and my healing meditations, my fragile body slowly began to become stronger and more flexible. I achieved a level of well-being I had not known before. I felt healthier than I had ever been. I also began to practice Ayurveda on others and saw how it transformed their life and their well-being.

It was 1994, at the age of 32, when I experienced a very clear vision. I was sitting in meditation when a surge of energy flowed through me that made my heart beat faster. The vision was both visual and auditory, though I have no doubt that only I could see and hear it. When it was over, it was clear what I was supposed to do. My dharma (higher purpose) was continuing to unfold, and I was being called upon to begin to build a profession for Ayurveda in the United States. The vision included a college where students could study to become ayurvedic practitioners. It also included building other components of the infrastructure of the profession, such as a State and National Association for the ayurvedic profession. When I told my wife she said, "Are you crazy, do you have any idea how much work you are talking about?!" I said, "How hard could it be? I'll start by holding classes at our home." We had our garage remodeled into my office and it made a perfect classroom. She was supportive, even if she did think I was crazy. She seemed to know far better than me that I had no idea what I was getting myself into. I didn't think about it. I had decided to surrender years ago. In my mind, I had no choice. You don't receive a vision unless you are willing to surrender to it. You don't receive a vision unless you have within you the hidden ability to fulfill it. The journey unlocks the potential.

In the latter part of 1994 I began the planning for the College. My main teacher at that time was Dr. Subhash Ranadé who lived in Pune, India. He made frequent trips to my home, which was now in Grass Valley, California. With his blessings and those of Dr. David Frawley, I began to organize the curriculum while utilizing them to fill in gaps in my own knowledge. Dr. Ranadé brought me copies of the classical ayurvedic texts dating back thousands of years and I began to study them cover to cover, extracting out the most relevant subject matter, and incorporating it in the school's curriculum. In October of 1995, I opened the California College of Ayurveda. As I understand it, it was the first State-Approved program designed to train practitioners of Ayurveda outside of India. Twenty-two students attended the first class and most came back one weekend each month for the next 15 months to continue their study. Interest was so high that I began another course six months later with 28 more students. The school quickly outgrew my home and within a year I had leased a building for the College. Six months later, the College opened a clinic for its students to practice and begin providing ayurvedic health care to our local community. When the first class of students graduated in 1997, we began the California Association of Ayurvedic Medicine. And a year later, in conjunction with several other leaders in the profession (Wynn Werner, Cynthia Copple and Kumar Batra) began the National Ayurvedic Medical Association (NAMA).

What was it about Ayurveda that inspired me to dedicate my life to the development of the profession? Yes, I was guided by the Divine, but it was more than that. I had found what I had been looking for. I had found the cause of disease and suffering. Think about it. If you had found the cause of heart disease, cancer and other conditions, would you feel compelled to share that knowledge? I knew that I would be devoting the rest of my life to the propagation of Ayurveda - for my own health and for all of humanity.

I have written two textbooks on the science of Ayurveda, Principles of

Ayurvedic Medicine and Clinical Ayurvedic Medicine. Today, I embark on writing my first book for you. As I sit down, I realize that, while my hands are moving and I appear to be typing this book, the words and the knowledge that is flowing onto these pages are not my own. They are the words and the knowledge of the Divine. The most I can do is surrender my hands and pray that they may be used to bring greater health and peace of mind to all who choose to read this book.

LESSON 1: THE CAUSE OF DISEASE AND SUFFERING

Only when the true cause of one's suffering is known does the path to healing become clear

Imagine what life would be like if you absolutely knew why you suffered physically and emotionally. Now imagine if you knew what to do in order to remove the cause. Would you try to remove it? Since the beginning of time, humanity has yearned to exist without suffering - to enjoy life and not be plagued by the struggles that attach themselves to daily experience. This has been the quest of Ayurveda and yoga for more than 5000 years. Ayurveda is the science of how to create optimal health. Yoga is the science of how to attain peace of mind. Together, Ayurveda and yoga, with roots in the soil of India, provide a complete set of knowledge of how to attain these goals.

In my quest to understand the cause of disease and suffering, I came to know from the ancient textbooks that there is not one but three fundamental causes of disease and suffering. If removed, each person is assured of a maximum life span. The three fundamental causes of disease are:

- The Misuse of the Senses
- The Failure of the Intellect
- Time

The Misuse of the Senses

The five senses of the body are like portals or gateways into the body, mind and consciousness. If a person takes in that which is harmonious, they will receive the nutrients and impressions that support life. If a person takes in that which is disharmonious, the body and mind will suffer. The challenge, of course, is to know what is harmonious and what is disharmonious.

In many ways, we are much like plants. If a plant lives in the right environment and receives all of the proper nutrients, has healthy soil, proper sunlight and is growing in the right temperature, it will attain a deep rich color and have lots of blossoms. If it does not, it may still survive, but it will not thrive and reach its full potential of beauty. We are much the same. Our environment is what we take in through the five senses: food, sights, sounds, smells and touch. If our environment is ideal, each of us will attain a deep, rich color and fully blossom into a healthy, whole and joyous human being. If not, we may still survive but our well-being will be significantly compromised and there is no way we can reach our full potential.

It is easy to understand how what you take in through the mouth will affect your well-being. Naturally, some foods are more nutritious than others. A diet that consists primarily of cupcakes and candy will not sustain most people while a diet of fruits and vegetables will lead to general health. Ayurveda takes this knowledge much further and is able to predict which fruits and vegetables are best for you and why. This is a major breakthrough. Some people's bodies respond better than others do to leafy greens. The same is true of root vegetables. Even within those categories, Ayurveda reveals more specific information. Carrots can be healthier for one person and potatoes for another. An ayurvedic food program tells you which vegetables, grains, nuts, seeds, dairy, oils and spices are healthiest for you and which will cause imbalances and suffering.

The same principles are true for the use of your other four senses. Sights, sounds, smells and touch can either support your health or contribute to sickness and suffering. We have all heard the old adage, "you are what you eat". This is only partially true. Ayurveda teaches that we are also what we see, hear, smell and touch.

The science of Ayurveda explores how we use our senses in order to understand how our actions have contributed to our diseases and how we can use them differently to support healing. After all, if the misuse of the senses is powerful enough to alter the body's physiology and create illness, then proper use of the senses must be powerful enough to again alter the body's physiology and support healing. Ayurveda is the science of how to effectively use diet and herbs, visual images and colors, music and words, and aromatherapy and massage to create within the body the optimum environment for healing to take place.

There is no one right way to use the senses. We are all unique. Nothing is right for everyone and everything is right for someone. Ayurveda is the science of learning what is right for you!

The Failure of the Intellect

How many things do you already know - that if you did – you would be healthier or happier than you are right now? For almost everyone, there is a long list. Most people know that if they went to bed earlier, they would feel less tired during the day. Some know that if they woke up earlier and had a relaxed morning that included some exercise and time for reflection, they would have a better disposition throughout the day. Almost everyone knows that if they gave up sugar or ate less fast food, they would be healthier. Yet, in spite of knowledge, choices are often made to act in a manner that is contradictory to the goals of health and well-being. This is an important part of what is meant by "The Failure of the Intellect."

The question arises as to why it is so difficult to implement what we know is best for us? The answer is not an easy one to understand. It is found within the philosophies that underlie Ayurveda, known as Sankhya and Vedanta. Put simply, there is a part of us that is in fear of change and in fear of reaching our physical or emotional potential. The status quo, the way things are now, is the preferred way of being for our ego. Our ego is attached to how we act now, not how we'd like to act or how we know deep inside that we should act in order to be healthy. That makes change very difficult because the ego controls our ordinary way of being and perceives change as its own death.

The role of the intellect is to process what we experience and make choices based on understanding. Our intellect has connections to both our ego and to our higher self, or soul. Each is providing different information for the intellect to consider before making any choice. The ego experiences the world through the senses. The senses provide the intellect with information about which of our choices will bring greater pleasure and avoid the most suffering. The ego and the senses work together and, from their perspective, the world and our choices are really quite black or white, pleasure or pain. If all we were was our ego, our choices would always be based on the pursuit of pleasure and its related enticements: power and money. Or, perhaps more simply, we would choose dessert over vegetables.

However, secondary input comes to the intellect from the higher self, or soul. The purpose of this input is to provide information about which choice would bring about the greatest harmony and well-being. The soul's interest is not in pleasure and pain but in the pursuit of the highest ideals. From the Vedic perspective, the soul's highest ideal is enlightenment or liberation from the cycle of birth and death. From a Judeo-Christian perspective, the soul's highest ideal is in entering the kingdom of heaven. Either way, following the soul's direction leads a person to make choices that go beyond the interests of short-term pleasures.

But, whom do we listen to most often, the soul's voice or the voice of the senses / ego? The answer, of course, is the ego. This is because the ego speaks loudly while the soul speaks in whispers. Few people ever clearly hear the whispering of their soul. We live in a highly stimulating sensory world. The noise created by the party being thrown for us every day makes it difficult to hear the soul's voice. Televisions, radios, Ipods, advertisements, road and city noise, and even talking and socializing, all create a web of sensory dramas that captivates the mind and prevents the whispers of the soul from being heard. Without soul awareness we perceive ourselves only as a body and mind. And with this limited perception, it is no wonder that we live each day in the pursuit of pleasure. Life becomes all about the pursuit of wealth, power and the next sensory high. The inability to hear the soul's voice gave birth to the adage, "who ever dies with the most toys wins."

In order to hear the whispers of the soul and empower the intellect to make harmonious choices, it is important for each of us to cultivate a proper life-style; one that brings quiet to the disturbances of the mind. Through taking quiet walks and the practices of meditation and yoga, the mind becomes calm and the voice of the soul can be heard. When a person first hears their soul's voice, the course of their life is changed forever. From a Vedic perspective, it is through the soul that the Divine communicates with us. Soul awareness is Divine awareness and with it, each person is empowered to control their senses and act in a manner that brings about peace of mind and optimal health.

Time

Time is the great equalizer. There will come a time when each of us will go through our transition from this life into that great mystery we call death. For those who live long enough, the process of time leads to gradual decay and this decay hastens the transition. But time is not necessarily a fixed concept. There are two kinds of time. One is linear and the other is biological. Both are based on motion.

Linear time is the measure of seconds, minutes, hours, days and years. We can do little to slow down the process of linear time. Linear time is based on the rotation of the earth around its axis and around the sun. Unless a person is powerful enough to stop celestial motion, time will pass and each person's age will be measured.

Biological time, however, is much more interesting. Biological time is the aging process. Biological time speeds up and slows down in accordance with our own personal motion. The faster we move, the faster we age. In Western terms, this is most similar to the concept of stress. The busier we become, the more stress we are under, the greater the toll on the body. Stress leads to cellular oxidation, which slowly damages and ages the cells of our body. Interestingly, rather than addressing the cause, many people turn to antioxidant pills in order to treat the symptom.

We live busy lives. Between work, family and ourselves, most people are moving all the time. Add to that the stress of the commute to and from work and jetlag from travel between time zones, and the body is under a great amount of stress. The busier and more hectic life becomes, the faster the body breaks down. However, it is not the motion of the body that is the most important component generating biological time. The real culprit is the movement of the mind.

The faster the mind moves the faster the body ages. When the mind moves, it moves into the future or into the past. In the future, the mind is busy planning or worrying. In the past, it is busy reflecting or regretting. Rarely does the mind sustain itself in the present moment. The movement of the mind generates thoughts and feelings that cause each person to get caught up in the dramas of life. The more the mind gets caught up in drama, the greater the stress and the faster the aging of the body. In order to stop aging, we must stop time. In order to stop time, we must stop the mind and come into the present moment. When we do this, biological time stands still. While stopping the mind completely may not be a practical goal for most people, the lesson is clear. Slowing down our lives, and especially our mind, is important if we want greater health and well-being. Ayurveda and yoga use the tool of meditation to accomplish this goal. Ordinary meditation accomplishes this goal while a person is sitting in meditation. The goal of Ayurveda is to turn each and every action into a form of meditation by being fully conscious and aware while taking each action. An ayurvedic lifestyle is a lifestyle of present moment consciousness.

In the present moment, there is nothing but perfection. Think about it: in this moment, is anything really wrong? Is there anything to worry about or be angry about? Probably not. Anger occurs when the mind is in the past. Worry occurs when the mind is focused on the future. In the present moment, all is well. With this realization, the mind and body are filled with the feelings that bring about healing: joy, love and bliss. There is no stress and the body functions optimally without any obstructions. A wounded body heals. A healthy body remains well. This is the fruit of stillness.

In order to slow down the mind, we must become more conscious of every action. In other words, when you are at work, think of nothing but work. When you are with your family, think of nothing but your family. Be present where you are and with what you are doing. There is an old quip that goes something like this. Don't be like the preacher who when preaching is thinking about making love to his wife and when he's making love to his wife is thinking about preaching. He wasn't a very good preacher or a very good husband. Thoughts are very distracting. When you are in the present you will become absorbed in the task at hand and in doing so, your mind will calm down and you will experience peace. In the Buddhist tradition, this has simply been called Mindfulness, the meditation of life.

Ayurveda, Stress and the Cause of Disease

Western science has well documented the effects of stress on the body. Many scientists and researchers are convinced that stress is the single most important cause of chronic disease. The role of stress was first brought into the limelight by Hans Selye in his book, "The Stress of Life" written in the 1950's. A pioneer in the field of mind-body medicine, his work has been built upon by many others since then and has given rise to the field of medicine known today as psycho-neuro-immunology. This field of medicine studies the interaction between the mind, the nervous system and the immune system. It is the study of how our thoughts and feelings affect our physiology. Essentially, it boils down to this: When you are under stress, your mind becomes more negative and your physiology becomes abnormal resulting in physical and mental disease. Continued stress then slows down or inhibits the healing process.

The mechanisms of the malfunctions are quite complex and varied but involve the dysfunction of most of the major organs of the body. Important physiological abnormalities secondary to stress include:

- The sympathetic nervous system becomes activated resulting in a faster heart rate, blood vessel constriction (a factor in hypertension and heart disease) and other changes that are factors that make it difficult to relax.

- The adrenal gland secretes more adrenalin. This helps activate the sympathetic nervous system.

- The adrenal gland secretes more cortisol at first and less as a person becomes exhausted. Cortisol is involved in blood sugar regulation and is an important hormone that regulates the immune system. Abnormal function is a part of most chronic stress diseases such as autoimmune disorders. Cortisol level abnormalities have also been implicated as a factor in obesity.

- Changes in brain biochemistry: Alterations of neurotransmitter levels affect mood.

- Immune factors decrease in the blood: Special proteins called Interleukins become less active. These are involved in prevention of viral infections and cancers.

Ayurveda would agree that stress is a significant cause of disease. In fact, Ayurveda is the science of what is stressful for an individual. While the proper use of the senses creates a stress-free environment, the misuse of the senses creates stress. In addition, the movement of the mind is another form of stress. When the mind gets caught up in the dramas of daily living, the physiology of the body becomes unhealthy. As this occurs, the door to disease opens. If the stress levels are too high, the protective factors of the body are depleted and illness occurs. Ayurveda and its sister science, yoga, are paths that lead to a stress-free existence and in doing so support the healing processes of the body.

Personal Reflections

Why did I become sick? What was the cause of my illness? It is never easy to pinpoint the cause of illness. We can only look at our lifestyle for clues. I was 25 years old when I became crippled by the autoimmune disease. By all rights, I should have been near the peak of my good health. In examining my lifestyle I can see several contributing factors that came into play that contributed to my condition. First, there are those that have to do with misusing my senses. My diet was not very good. It wasn't bad by most middle American standards but it really wasn't good. I had been a college student for seven years after all and even before that it wasn't great, having grown up on fast foods and indulging excessively in cookies and ice cream. As an undergraduate I drank what today I would consider a lot of alcohol. I also smoked a good deal of marijuana and indulged from time to time in everything from cocaine to LSD. After many late nights I found myself at Perkins, our local 24-hour restaurant eating both breakfast and lunch at the same time. Even in Chiropractic school with my diet vastly improving, I found myself at happy hour drinking Margaritas and making dinner of the Mexican snack foods. I knew better but my actions were lagging behind my knowledge and my intellect failed me. I compounded the situation by staying up late at night to party and not getting enough sleep. Time and motion contributed as well. My mind moved very fast and that created a lot of stress. I was intensely focused on my school work when I wasn't out partying to try to relax. I worried about exams and that drove me even harder. All of this accumulated throughout the years, but it was near graduation that my body broke down. Graduating was stressful! I found myself deep in education debt and feeling the stress of the transition from student to grown-up. I knew how to be a student. I didn't know how to be a grown-up. Piling on to the stress was the reality that my parents, who divorced when I was 16 years old and were in a bitter and angry stage of their post-divorce relationship, were about to collide at my graduation ceremony. Well, the combination of misusing my senses, the failure of my intellect and the motion of my mind eventually broke the back of my immune system. My body had become too weak from the abuse to withstand the assault and it broke down.

Now it can be argued that others have had to endure worse and that their bodies did not break down. Perhaps, but each person responds to stress differently. Vedic philosophy teaches that this is a result of a person's karma. Past actions set the stage for current suffering. Sometimes those actions are obvious and sometimes they are not.

Later, during the back injury, it was apparent that I was not on my proper path of service. I was serving through Chiropractic but my higher Self was not satisfied and needed to go deeper. The dichotomy between my Chiropractic service (reducing pain and suffering) and the service I was meant to do (removing the cause of pain and suffering) created yet another schism in my mind.

My back injury and the immune system disorder that left me with Chronic Fatigue Syndrome were guideposts to help me get back on track. Of course, reading the signs and acting on them are quite different. It took a lot of suffering before I yielded and surrendered.

Exercise: Start a Healing Your Life Journal

- Write down five examples of how you misuse your senses on a weekly basis.

- Make a list of five things that you already know you could do to improve your well-being but are not currently doing.

- Write down the aspects of your life that are out of harmony and cause stress. When you are done, label each one either "Future", "Past" or "Present Moment", depending upon which timeframe is

LESSON 2: PATIENCE

Water gently flows over the rocks and after
thousands of years a canyon is formed.

We do not push the wind; it is the wind that pushes us. Life moves each person forward at just the right pace to stimulate continued learning and growth. There is little each person can do to rush the process. The most we can do is to become a more conscious participant.

When faced with the challenge of creating new behaviors, some approach the challenge head on and work hard, only to eventually burn out through the struggle and finally give up. Others get overwhelmed quickly and do not make much progress before realizing that the task is just too daunting. They too give up. Still others see what it is that needs to get done, think it is a good idea but never get started from a lack of motivation. Perceiving oneself as having failed only makes the situation worse and so, rather than try again, most people distract themselves so that they do not have to face the challenge.

As you read more and more about Ayurveda, you will see that it brings you face to face with your current lifestyle choices and asks you to compare them to an ideal. When doing so, we inevitably fall short, for who among us is so pure and so holy that we have no faults. Indeed, that is a rare individual. When looking into the mirror of Ayurveda, most people begin to see many areas that are in need of improvement and at the same time offer great opportunities for growth and healing. Without patience though, overwhelm, burnout or inertia will get the best of us.

Patience requires a proper perspective. Transforming your lifestyle is a journey. It is not reasonable to expect that you will be able to do everything that can be done to improve your health and well-being or even make a large number of changes quickly. Even small, simple changes can make a profound difference in how you feel. In fact, progress on the path of Ayurveda is really just making a series of small, profound changes.

Our most basic behaviors come from a place deep inside that Ayurveda refers to as our consciousness. Change at the level of consciousness is both the most profound and the most difficult. Even a simple change at this level of our being ripples out into every aspect of our experience of life. Imagine how your life might change if you successfully made only the one change that you already know you need to make. How does the smoker's life change when they give up cigarettes or the alcoholic's life when they give up drinking?

A person who has patience accepts that there may be periods of challenge and even what some would call failure. However, with patience, there is no failure until you give up. In other words, to the smoker with patience who gives up cigarettes for a month and then goes back, the commitment to transformation has not changed. Soon, he or she will quit smoking again. It may take a year or more to give up the habit but with patience comes eventual success. This is true for changing any habit.

The Cake Metaphor for Patience

One day you decide that you would really like to eat cake. You've heard that it tastes great. So you get started taking the actions a person takes who wants to taste cake. You gather the ingredients and mix them together according to the recipe and place the batter into the oven. If you don't have patience, then after a few minutes you take it out and see that it is still flat and unappetizing. Seeing this perhaps you give up. However, if you are patient you keep it in the oven and soon the dough rises and the batter transforms itself into a cake. You taste it and delight in the transformation.

The batter is your current state of consciousness, your current body and mind. You begin to take the actions that create transformation. If you expect transformation to happen quickly, you are likely to be disappointed. With patience though, your actions will yield a new state of consciousness, a new body and mind and you will experience the joy of greater well-being.

The Metaphor of the Lotus Flower

The lotus flower grows slowly and each petal opens in its own time. Likewise, one's consciousness, body and mind is transformed at his or her own pace. If you force open a flower, you pull off the petals and more harm is done than good. Even good intentions can cause harm when actions are taken without wisdom. If you are patient, the full beauty of the flower will reveal itself in the proper time. Don't pull too hard on your own petals. If you do, rather than opening into the brilliant flower that you are, you will injure yourself physically or emotionally. Allow yourself to bloom naturally.

Personal Reflections

When I was a young boy, my mother and father used to say to me, "Think before you speak." I was often impulsive and I would do and say things that were not well thought out.

As a very young boy, about 7 years old, I had a speech impediment. I stuttered, stammered and spoke with a lisp. Often, I just could not get the next word out. It must have run in my family, because my father did as well when he was a child. While he overcame his impediment through singing and placing marbles in his mouth when he spoke (it must have slowed him down), I received a combination of speech therapy and my father's reminders to slow down. While speech therapy must have helped a bit, it was slowing down that really made the big difference. I relaxed and my thoughts settled. Then, the words came out with no problem. It was a process of developing patience.

As I study my own speech processes, I observe how my thoughts appear to arise from my subconscious mind, enter into my conscious mind for processing and then work their way out my mouth. The problem for me with speaking was that thoughts appeared to move from my subconscious directly to my mouth without the proper processing. The thought was half-baked as it was trying to come out my mouth and I would stutter and stammer. Once it started, my attention went to my problem and that just made the problem worse.

In order to correct the problem I had to begin to learn patience. This began with acceptance and a certain amount of surrender. I had to first accept that I had a problem. Now of course, that was obvious but, by acceptance and surrender, I mean that I had to stop wrestling with the problem, stop believing that with greater focus and effort I could just push through it. That just wasn't going to happen. I had to do the opposite. I had to slow down and relax. I had to let the words form in my mind so that I knew what I wanted to say, and then they could form in my mouth. I had to think before I spoke. As time went on, my speech improved more and more. As my conscious and subconscious mind began to communicate effectively with each other, my conscious thought process began to occur much more rapidly and the delay in my responses became more and more socially appropriate.

Today, I am considered to be a very good public speaker. People often remark that I speak clearly and that my talks are well thought out. Even today, as I speak to audiences or in the classroom, I am conscious of my thought processes working out the details of what I am about to say before I say it. This all happens very quickly and, to the audience, I simply appear thoughtful, thinking before I speak.

Some people are by nature very patient. For me, patience had to be learned and then learned again and again. My nature is to act quickly. The story I just told you is one of the first lessons in patience I received.

Exercise: Patience

Find a quiet place out in nature, a park is perfect, but a quiet street can work too. Choose a point about 100 yards away. Walk toward it slowly; one small step at a time. As you walk, allow yourself to feel each foot meeting the ground. Keep your eyes looking about five yards in front of you toward the ground. You may struggle at first with the slow pace. As you walk forward, observe your breath going in and out. Keep your attention on your breath and your feet. If any feelings arise (frustration, anxiety), simply observe them. Do not process the feeling, just notice it and let it go. There are two parts to your experience: there is the feeling and there is the part of you that is observing the feeling. Focus on the part of you that is observing how you feel rather than the feeling itself. This part of you is at peace and may even be amused at the other part. Smile as you notice the anxiety or the frustration. If you do this, the feeling will diminish. Continue to move forward one small step at a time while remaining focused on your breath. You will arrive at your destination. Let this exercise be a metaphor for the longer and more arduous journey of achieving optimal health and peace of mind.

LESSON 3: THE PRIMORDIAL CAUSE OF DISEASE

Who is that I see in the mirror? Whose thoughts flow through this mind? Is that really me?

The mind, caught up in the dramas of life, can not accurately perceive the true nature of who we are. Rather, what we see and therefore believe is that we are limited to this body and mind, to this state of health and these thoughts and feelings. But is that who we really are? Few of us have the ability to accurately perceive ourselves. What we see is a highly distorted image and with that vision, we get caught in the drama of self-perception. This is drama that limits our perception and our potential inevitably leading to suffering. To the degree that we can successfully escape this drama, expand our perceptions and our potential, is the degree to which we take control over our lives, become the master of our ego and ultimately find both peace of mind and perfect health. In order to accomplish this, we must practice self-study.

Self-study—the willingness to observe and examine one's actions, motivations and existence is rarely easy, as a close look often reveals what we don't want to see: imperfection. If you find yourself avoiding self-study, it may comfort you to know that you are not alone. Most people would prefer to walk barefoot over broken glass than sit still and look within. But what if you did look within, beyond the drama, the pain and the suffering, what would you see? Supposing I told you that you would look upon infinite beauty, blissful peace and unlimited potential and possibility. Indeed, this is what the ancient teachers of Ayurveda and yoga taught and it is the ultimate secret to good health as well.

In order to have this vision, it is necessary to become quiet and still within. In order to sustain that vision, it is necessary to bring that stillness into every action. This is stillness in action and it is the key to perfect health.

But what would you see? What lies even beyond the perceptions of infinite beauty, blissful peace and unlimited potential and possibility? The simple answer is The Divine. This is our true nature and forgetting this is the primordial cause of all disease and suffering. Realizing this opens up the flood gates allowing tremendous energy and power to flow through this creation we call our bodies and minds. This power put to use can do anything within the laws of nature. It can help us control our senses, master our ego and certainly bring about healing and peace of mind. However, many people abuse this power and put it to use in the pursuit of riches and power. These pursuits only lead to eventual blindness once again and the individual gets lost in the world and once again suffers until he or she loses what matters most, health and peace of mind.

Forgetting our true nature as Divine beings is the reason why we misuse our senses. It is why the intellect fails us and it is why we get caught up in the dramas that generate biological time. It is the source of all suffering. If we are not Divine beings then what are we? We are our bodies and our minds, our thoughts and our dramas. If this is true, then no wonder we suffer.

The process of forgetting begins as soon as we are conceived and becomes more and more complete as we become more and more established in our ego and sensory self. Shortly after birth, the door to our Divine memory closes. As we forget our true nature as Divine, we perceive ourselves more and more to be our body and mind and we come to know the world and the nature of existence only through our senses. The pursuit of pleasure and the avoidance of pain become the largest part of the meaning of life. Caught up in the ego and the experience of the mind, we begin to identify ourselves by what makes us different from everyone else. That process usually begins with: I am a child. I am my name. I am a boy or I am a girl. It continues on and we say: I am a white person or a black person. I am a big person or a small person. I am a person with long hair or short hair. I am a heavy or thin person. I am athletic or intellectual. I am a conservative or a liberal. You can see how it happens. As we grow up and reach our early adult years, we become more and more individualized and separated from the whole in an effort to define our uniqueness and become self (ego) confident. Through the ego, we create a web of illusion about ourselves that dominates our experience and we accept it as real. Through this process we become less Self (Divine / soul) confident. The process of yoga is the process of peeling away the layers of illusion until what is left is an awareness of our true natures as Divine Spirit. As we go through that process, Ayurveda exists to keep us healthy so that we can continue our spiritual work. The role of Ayurveda is to teach us how to successfully manage the illusion without getting caught up in it. The role of yoga is to teach us how to transcend the illusion.

The journey of Ayurveda and yoga is the journey of healing ourselves physically, emotionally and spiritually. What begins with looking at oneself and examining one's challenges ends with Self-realization and the awareness of Divine unity in all creation. It is the journey of a thousand miles and it begins with the first step.

Personal Reflections

Coming to know my own true nature has been a gradual process of remembering and forgetting again and again. Each time I remember, I feel a surge of peace, love and joy that is difficult to put into words. Then, life and drama creep in and I forget as I get caught up in the roller coaster of emotion and self-importance. Suffering has been my greatest teacher in this respect. Fortunately, today I don't have to suffer as much as I used to. As my mind drifts into worldly dramas, I never seem to drift too far anymore. I am tethered to the memory through my spiritual practices. Through creating altars, meditating, practicing and teaching yoga and Ayurveda, I am constantly reminded of my True Nature and this provides me with the power to gain greater mastery over my senses and my ego. While I am by no means at the end of my journey and able to sustain my awareness at all moments, I am making steady progress. And, I am reminded that even the journey is an illusion of drama and in that realization, I rest in peace.

Exercise: Self-Study: Who Am I?

- Find a peaceful quiet place
- Bring a pencil and paper
- Write down as many ideas about who you are as possible.
- Complete the sentence, I am.......
- Let yourself explore all your self definitions and identifications
- Write as many "I am" statements as come to mind. Include all physical, emotional and spiritual ideas of who you are. Include all labels that you identify with.
- When your list is complete, turn those statements around into "I am NOT ..... each of those ideas. Read them out loud.
- Sit quietly and reflect on who you are now that you have let go of each identification.
- Who are you?
- Take time to write in your journal about your experience with this exercise. Try not to judge your experience. Let it be pure and true.

LESSON 4: QUALITIES, ELEMENTS AND THE THREE DOSHAS

Beyond the atom, beyond the subatomic particle, lie the qualities of existence waiting to combine and take form.

According to the philosophy of Ayurveda and yoga, we are all manifestations of Divine potentials. In this sense, we all emerge from the same ocean of pure consciousness and within each of us lies all of the knowledge of pure existence. While on this level we are all truly One, when the body and mind form, we become a unique expression of that potential. While from a philosophical and spiritual perspective the body and mind are a transient illusion sure to one day go back to the dust from which it came, knowledge of the illusion is essential to being able to properly care for ourselves and reduce illness and suffering.

Central to the practices of Ayurveda is the knowledge of the five elements and the three doshas. The five elements are our most basic building blocks. The three doshas are the fundamental biological energies governing the functions of the body and mind and are called vata, pitta and kapha.

Each of us has a unique balance of the five elements and the three doshas and this balance is called our constitution. Our constitution is determined at the moment of conception and is with us for the rest of our lives. It determines what we are naturally attracted to and what will cause us to become out of balance, sick and diseased. Knowledge of our constitution is fundamental to staying healthy.

Each of us is unique. No two people were ever created with the same constitution. For this reason, there is no one diet or lifestyle program that meets everyone's needs. Disturbances in the natural balance of these three energies result in suffering in the body and mind. The goal of ayurvedic treatment is to restore the natural, healthy balance of the doshas—to return a person to the balance present at conception. When the doshas are in their proper balance, the physical body has the best chance of healing itself and reaching its full potential.

A person who understands the doshic nature of their constitution and the doshic nature of any imbalances present has the information at hand to take the proper actions to restore their natural balance. Ayurveda utilizes lifestyle, diet, herbs and sensory therapies (color therapy, aroma therapy, sound therapy and massage therapy) as the basic tools to restore balance. Ayurveda utilizes all aspects of yoga to deepen the healing process, including breathing practices, asanas (yoga postures) and meditation. These practices applied to the healing process are collectively called Ayurvedic Yoga Therapy.

The Five Elements

When you think of the five elements, think of the most basic building blocks of matter. In the West, we are used to thinking of the basic building blocks as being atoms. Even more basic are the electrons, protons and neutrons. Subatomic particles become even more basic than that. At the subatomic level, the idea of a building block being a solid begins to break down. At that level, a particle has a lot in common with a wave of energy. As the scientific mind goes deeper, the physical concepts of matter disappear altogether. The origins of matter become mathematical equations of probability. A probability could be called an idea that has a chance of manifesting into form. The field of probabilities is the ocean of primordial soup from which all matter comes into existence. Vedic science calls this primordial soup, prakruti. The field is immense, it is infinite and within it exist all possibilities. From it, probabilities emerge and of those probabilities, some manifest. Exactly how that occurs remains a mystery.

The ayurvedic concept of the basic building blocks of matter is very similar to that found in higher mathematics and physics. A building block is an idea. All of creation is built from five ideas. The five ideas are summarized as the five elements. Each element, however, is more than it appears to be on the surface. It is a poetic key to existence itself.

Air

Air is the idea of motion. Motion begins as a possibility, evolves to a probability and emerges into the world as all of the physical forces in the universe that have the capacity to move things. This includes all of the known and unknown forces such as magnetism, gravity, thermodynamics and propulsion, as well as celestial forces such as the effect of the moon on the tides. All are a function of the idea of air. In the body, air is responsible for the motion we see in nerve impulses, circulation and the movement of the joints. In the mind, air moves our thoughts. On the cellular level, air is responsible for cytoplasmic circulation and the movement of oxygen and nutrients into the cell and of carbon dioxide and waste out of the cell. On the atomic level, the concept of air moves the subatomic particles. Air is responsible for the frequency of vibrations found at the intersection of matter and energy and in the energy itself. When air is mentioned in Ayurveda, it means much more than the wind or the air we breathe. It is a fundamental concept of life. It is a building block. Nothing can move if there is no air. Nothing can move if there is no force to move it. All forces of the universe are aspects of air.

The more air you have in your constitution, the faster your mind and body move.

Fire

Fire, as an idea, represents heat, light and the power of transformation. Fire is the building block of all metabolic transformations in the universe. These transformations give off light and heat. The sun is the celestial fire. Its metabolic reactions produce the heat that fuels our lives. Metabolic reactions also generate light. The chemical reactions of the sun produce the light we see every day. The electrochemical reactions of the light bulb also generate light. In the body, metabolic and electrochemical reactions are constantly taking place. These reactions also produce light. Although this light is too faint for the ordinary human eye to perceive, it can be "seen" through instrumentation. Many refer to this light as the aura. In the mind, the subtle biochemical reactions that create understanding also produce a type of light. The greater the understanding, the brighter the light. The illumination of the mind leads to clear perception and dispels the darkness of ignorance.

The more fire you have in your constitution, the warmer your body,
the stronger your digestion and the sharper your mind.

Water

Water is the idea of cohesion. As a fundamental building block of nature, water is the cohesive principle that holds everything together, even the atoms that make up a molecule. It is a centrifugal force pulling toward the center. Water clings to the idea of stability like a droplet of rain that hangs from a gutter. Even as it finally falls, it holds itself together, until impacted by the force of the ground.

The concept of water is perceived in nature as fluid. The cohesive force holds things together but only loosely. So, it can be moved by the mobile forces of nature (air). When it does move, the cohesive quality causes it to move in a slow, graceful, flowing manner. Thus, anything that moves in a slow, flowing manner can be said to contain water, even oil. In the body, water is the plasma, the urine, the saliva, the oil secretions, the fluid that surrounds each cell, and the fluid inside the cell. In the mind, the cohesive quality is responsible for deep feelings and attachment. It creates the tendency to cling to people and things. Some emotions have a water nature. These move in a flowing manner as well. Watery emotions include love, empathy and compassion.

The more water you have in your constitution, the more
you are likely to attach yourself to people, things or ideas.

Earth

Earth is the idea of solidity. As a fundamental building block of nature, earth is found in all that is solid. It is denser than water and more difficult to move. The structure of the universe is predicated on the idea of earth. Without it, there is no structure for energy to flow through. Earth makes up the solid matter of the planets and all that is solid on this planet, but earth is much more. In the body, earth makes up all of the solid structures such as bones, muscles, hair and organs. On a subtler level, the cell membrane is made up of earth. So are the intracellular organelles, such as the mitochondria and ribosomes. Even the DNA found in the nucleus of the cell is an expression of the earth element.

Go smaller still and the solid structures of an atom are made up of earth. In the mind, earth gives structure to ideas.

The more earth you have in your constitution,
the denser your body, and the more fixed you become in your ideas and beliefs.

Ether

Ether is the idea of empty space. As a fundamental building block of nature, ether is the most subtle of all. On the cosmic level, ether is the field of existence from which all else emerges. It is the field of possibilities and probabilities. On a more physical level, ether is the space that exists between things and that which connects everything together. In the body, ether is expressed as empty space. Empty space is not really empty in the body because it is immediately filled up by the other elements. Thus, ether is the space that the other elements fill. If ether increases in the body, it damages the other elements, essentially erasing them, and causes the elemental structure of the body to break down. Ether is also the field of the mind; the place where ideas (possibilities) emerge.

The more ether you have in your constitution, the more subtle your awareness and
the more possibilities you will remain open to.

Vedic knowledge teaches that all of creation comes from the cosmic field of unlimited possibilities (ether). The movement (air) of some of these possibilities into probabilities makes them real on the subtlest physical levels. Some of these probabilities are then birthed into physical existence. The process of transformation (fire) from a possibility to a probability and a probability into manifestation is a metabolic (fire) process that in turn generates heat and light. The force of cohesion (water) sustains and nourishes that which has manifested. When that which has manifested takes a solid, stable form (earth), it becomes most easily observable. Thus, we see that all of creation comes from the idea of ether, and all elements of creation manifest within the idea of earth.

Thousands of years ago, the ancient rishis of India described the origins of creation. Their description was not religious but scientific. As modern science and higher mathematics have advanced, they are now beginning to understand quantum physics and string theory. These incredible sciences are taking the Western mind to the same field of possibilities explored by the ancient teachers of India and thus providing validation of the principles upon which Ayurveda and yoga are founded.

The Qualities of Nature

The ancient teachers taught that in order to fully understand the nature of any aspect of creation, including the five elements, it is necessary to understand it in terms of ten pairs of opposing qualities. All of nature is made of a combination of these qualities. The qualities of a substance can be said to be its unique code. Knowledge of the code allows a person to accurately predict how two substances will interact with each other. This knowledge makes treatment possible in Ayurveda. If the qualities of a disease are understood and the qualities of the medicines are understood, then the practitioner of Ayurveda has the information needed to prescribe medicines that antidote the qualities of the disease. This same principle is true for disease prevention. Knowledge of the qualities of a substance allows a person who understands the qualities inherent within themselves to make lifestyle choices (diet, aromas, colors, sounds and touch) that support well-being. What follows is a brief description of the ten pairs of opposing qualities and some common sense suggestions.

Warm and Cool

Everything in nature is warm or cool. Naturally there is a spectrum of how warm or how cool something is. The terms simply relate to which side of the midpoint a substance (food, person, color, etc.) falls on. For instance, some spices, like black pepper, are clearly hot. Other spices, like cumin, are hot, but not as hot. Some substances, like milk and watermelon, are cooling. Taking in those substances increases the warm or cool quality in a person.

Common Sense:

If you have a chill, drink a cup of warm, spicy tea.
If you are too warm, drink more milk and snack on watermelon.

Heavy or Light

Everything in nature is heavy or light. Cheeses, meats and flour are examples of things that are heavy. Fruits and vegetables are generally light. Taking in those substances increases the corresponding quality in the body and mind.

Common Sense:

If you want to lose weight, eat more fruits and vegetables.
If you are too light, eat more cheese and bread.

Moist or Dry

Everything in nature is moist or dry. Milk, oil and butter are naturally moist. Corn flour products and popcorn are very dry. Fresh bread is moister than toasted bread. Taking in one of these foods will increase the corresponding quality in the body and mind.

Common Sense:

Heal your dry skin by taking in more oils through your diet.
If your skin is too oily, eat more popcorn, corn tortillas and toasted breads.
Hold the butter!

Mobile or Stable

Everything in nature is mobile or stable. To be mobile means that it either generates motion or makes something easier to move. To be stable means that it increases stability or makes something more difficult to move. Caffeinated coffee and tea are good examples of mobile substances. They make the body and mind move faster. A stable substance is often a heavy one. Meats, grains and cheeses are considered stable. To take one of these substances increases the corresponding quality in the body and mind.

Common Sense:

*If your mind won't slow down, eat more meat,
bread and cheese and avoid coffee and tea.*

*If your mind is too sluggish, a cup of coffee or tea
might help and eat less meat, bread and cheese.*

Sharp or Dull

Some things in nature are sharp and some are dull. Taking in those qualities will increase these qualities within a person. A person's mind can be sharp or dull. So can their manner of speech. Spices are sharp and so is vinegar. Meats, soft cheeses and potatoes are dull. Taking in those substances increases the quality of the substance in the body and mind.

Common Sense:

*If the words that you use are too sharp,
drink more milk and eat more cream cheese.*

If your mind is too dull, increase your intake of spices and vinegar.

Hard or Soft

Some things in nature are hard and some are soft. A root, bark, grain or bone is harder than a piece of cheese, fruit or a cup of milk. Whole grain wheat is harder than white flour. Taking in foods or other substances that are hard or soft will increase the corresponding qualities in the body and mind.

Common Sense:

*If your body is too soft, eat less cheese, drink less milk and eat less white flour.
Instead take in more whole grains and eat more root vegetables.*

Gross or Subtle

Gross means large and obvious, whereas subtle is less noticeable. When someone gains weight, their body becomes larger and more obvious. When someone loses weight, they become less noticeable. Things that are gross are usually heavier and that which is subtle is usually lighter. Meats and grains are gross, whereas leafy greens and spices are more subtle. Taking in these substances increases their corresponding qualities in the body and mind.

Common Sense:

*If you are overweight and your body is too large,
eat more leafy vegetables and increase your spices.*

If you are underweight and your body is not very
noticeable, eat more meat and grains.

Dense or Flowing

Some things in nature are denser than others. As density increases, flow decreases. An example of a dense substance would be a slice of bread, meat or a baked potato. Fluids are the best examples of a flowing substance. Milk and orange juice, as well as oils, are good examples. Taking in those substances will increase the corresponding qualities in the body and mind.

Common Sense:

If you have too much mucous, reduce your intake of oils, milk and juices. If your
body or mind is too dense, reduce your intake of bread, meat and potatoes.

Rough or Smooth

Everything in nature is rough or smooth and taking in substances with those qualities will increase the corresponding qualities within our body and mind. Cream cheese is a good example of a smooth substance. So is pudding. Smooth substances generally have more oils and fat in them. An example of a rough substance is a raw vegetable. These substances usually have a very low fat content and high roughage.

Common Sense:

If your skin is too dry, eat more cream
cheese and pudding. Add more oil to your foods.

Cloudy or Clear

In order to appreciate the qualities of cloudy and clear, think about the mind. Some days it is cloudier than others. Some people have generally a clearer mind than others. Substances that are cloudy include milk, meat and cheese. Substances that are clear include most vegetables and fruits. By taking in these substances, we increase the corresponding quality in our body and mind.

Common Sense:

If your mind is cloudy, eat more fruits and
vegetables and avoid meat, milk and cheese.

The Five Elements and the Qualities

While the five elements have been described as ideas that are the building blocks of nature, they are also the carriers of the ten pairs of opposite qualities. In order to really understand what is meant by an element, it is useful to know what its qualities are. Since we are all made up of the five elements, the balance of these elements within us determines the qualities of our body and mind. Below is a chart of the five elements showing the ten qualities found in each of those elements.

Summary of the Five Elements and the
Ten Pairs of Opposing Qualities Found in Nature

Qualities	Ether	Air	Fire	Water	Earth
Warm/Cool	Cool	Cool	Warm	Cool	Cool
Heavy/Light	Light	Light	Light	Heavy	Heavy
Moist/Dry	Dry	Dry	Dry	Moist	Dry
Mobile/Stable	Mobile	Mobile	Mobile	Stable	Stable
Sharp/Dull	Dull	Sharp	Sharp	Dull	Dull
Hard/Soft	Soft	Hard	Hard	Soft	Hard
Gross/Subtle	Subtle	Subtle	Subtle	Gross	Gross
Dense/Flowing	Flowing	Flowing	Flowing	Flowing	Dense
Rough/Smooth	Smooth	Rough	Rough	Smooth	Rough
Cloudy/Clear	Clear	Clear	Clear	Cloudy	Cloudy

Introduction to the Three Doshas

The three doshas are at the heart of Ayurveda. They are the basic physiological energies that govern the functions of the body. Vata dosha, made up of air and ether, is the energy of motion and controls circulation, the movements of nerve impulses, the movement of thought and the movement of the joints. Pitta dosha, made up primarily of fire and a little water, controls metabolism and digestion. Kapha dosha, made up of earth and water, controls the structure of the body. Everybody has all three of the doshas within them. A person's constitution is their unique balance of these three doshas. There are infinite constitutions based upon the percentage of each dosha within a person. As a result, some people are more mobile, some are more metabolic and some are more structured. But everyone has some of each and no two people are exactly alike. The balance of the three doshas within you determines what you are naturally attracted to and what will cause you to become out of balance – sick and diseased.

In order to gain an appreciation of how these doshas impact our bodies and minds, it is important to understand them from the perspective of their qualities. Each consists of its own combination of the ten pairs of opposing qualities.

The table below shows the elemental makeup and the qualities of each dosha. If you have a predominance of one dosha in your makeup (of course you have all three to some extent), your body and mind will reflect the qualities of that dosha. Often there is one dominant dosha and varying amounts of the others. Sometimes two doshas are present in close to equal amounts. Occasionally we see people with all three doshas in an equal balance. Your ideal balance is the balance that was present at conception. From that moment onward, you are affected by your environment and the choices that you make. Your environment and your choices can disturb the proper balance and create symptoms of disease and suffering.

Summary of the Qualities of the Three Doshas

Qualities	Vata	Pitta	Kapha
Elements	Air and Ether	Fire (mostly) and Water (a little)	Water and Earth
Warm/Cool	Cold	Warm	Cold
Heavy/Light	Light	Light	Heavy
Moist/Dry	Dry	Moist (slightly)	Moist
Mobile/Stable	Mobile	*Mobile	Stable
Sharp/Dull	Sharp	Sharp	Dull
Hard/Soft	Hard	Hard	Soft
Gross/Subtle	Subtle	Subtle	Gross
Dense/Flowing	Flowing	Flowing	Dense
Rough/Smooth	Rough	Rough	Smooth
Cloudy/Clear	Clear	Clear	Cloudy

*Pitta dosha is categorized as mobile; however, it is only vata dosha, composed of air, that is truly mobile. Pitta's motion is generated by heat that agitates the principle of air. This is why fire never stands still and those with a pitta nature are quick to take action when necessary.

LESSON 5: KNOW YOUR CONSTITUTION

One's constitution is like one's birth certificate.
It tells of where you got your start in life.

Your body is made up of the five elements. These elements combine together to create the three doshas. The balance of the three doshas in your body controls both the structure and function of your body. The balance that was present at the moment of conception is your constitution. This is your perfect balance. When it is sustained, you remain well. Your constitution determines what type of an environment is ideal for you and what type will make you sick. Knowledge of your constitution can help you to create an environment that keeps you well. If you are sick, knowledge of the nature of the imbalance can help you to restore your natural balance and maximize your healing process.

It is important to understand that the qualities inherent in your constitution are your natural qualities. They do not necessarily represent how you look or feel today. Whether or not you express these qualities has a lot to do with your environment and your experiences in life. Your environment and past experiences alter how the three doshas express themselves. These alterations are reflective of imbalances in the body and can act like a mask over your true constitution. As you return to balance, your true constitution will become more observable.

Your Physical Features

Your physical features can tell you a lot about your constitution. They are a reflection of the elements that make up your physical nature and the qualities inherent within the elements. An ayurvedic practitioner is very observant of your qualities and has the experience to notice subtle influences. Still, you can observe many of your own qualities and in doing so, learn about your constitution.

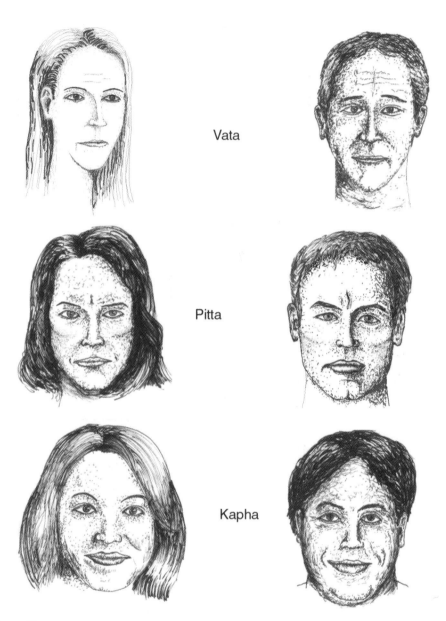

Vata

Pitta

Kapha

Your Face

On the face there are many features to observe. There is the angle of the jaw and shape of the face, there are the eyes, nose and lips as well as complexion. Below are six drawn faces that reveal the stereotypical characteristics of the three doshas.

The Shape of the Face and the Angle of the Jaw

If you look at these faces, you will notice that the ones at the top are narrow and longer. These are typical vata-type faces. They have the narrowest jaw line. The ones at the bottom are round. They have the widest jaw line. These are typical kapha faces. The faces in the middle have a strong jaw line and they have sharper features in general. The shape of the face is angular. These are typical pitta faces.

The Eyes

You will notice that the eyes in the vata drawings at the top are small. They are subtle and less noticeable. The eyes in the pitta faces in the middle are medium in size and they are deep set into the socket. This is a classic pitta feature and creates a fiery intensity in the eyes. People of pitta nature have a critical eye and examine the world very closely. The eyes in the kapha faces at the bottom are larger and watery. They are very attractive eyes and have a softer quality.

The Nose

It is the bridge of the nose that tells the most about its elemental makeup. The more air and ether, the narrower and more subtle it becomes. We see this in the vata nose bridge. The pitta nose bridge is moderate revealing that fire and water have a little more mass. The kapha nose bridge is wide. The earth and water in kapha have the greatest mass. The bridge of the nose is softer and fuller.

The Lips

The lips of the person with a vata face are thin. This again reflects the subtle and light qualities that result in the lack of mass found in air and ether. Those of a pitta face are moderate and those of a kapha face are full.

The Complexion

It is fire that creates the most dramatic color in the complexion; the greater the fire, the redder the complexion. Thus, a person with a pitta nature has a rosy or ruddy complexion. The lack of fire in a person with a vata nature creates a dusty or gray tone. In a kapha person it creates a pale tone.

The Hair

It is the earth element that gives the hair its fullness and thickness. Water gives it oiliness. Thus, a person with a kapha nature has thick, full hair that is moist or oily. A person with a pitta nature may also have oily hair as a result of the water element but their hair is fine. A person with a vata nature has dry, scanty hair. Because of its dryness, it feels coarse.

The Skin

It is the earth element that provides mass to the skin. Water makes it soft. Thus, the skin of a person with a kapha nature is thicker and softer than those of the other constitutional types. The skin of a person with a pitta nature is neither very thick nor thin but it is somewhat oily, owing to its slightly watery nature. The skin of a person with a vata nature, lacking in earth and water, is thinner and drier. This makes it rough as well.

The Bones (Arms, Fingers and Neck)

The earth element provides the bones with density and thickness. Thus, a person with a kapha nature has the thickest and densest bones. Their length is shorter relative to their circumference. In other words, the bones appear stocky. A person with a vata nature, having less earth in their nature, has thin or narrow bones. Their length is long when compared to the circumference. This allows for quick movements. The bones of those with a pitta nature are in-between, as fire and water are denser than air and ether but not as dense as water and earth.

The boney structure can be observed in many areas of the body. Ayurvedic practitioners often look at the arms between the elbow and the wrist. This is easiest to observe. Arms which are longer and narrower suggest more vata dosha in the constitution. Those which are shorter and thicker suggest more kapha. Those that are in-between suggest pitta.

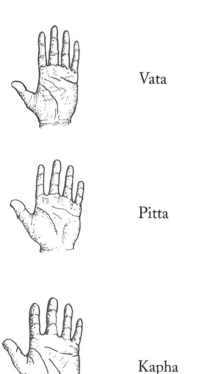

Vata

Pitta

Kapha

The boney structure of the body can also be observed in the neck. When observing the neck, you are actually observing the length provided by the vertebrae. The circumference is provided primarily by the musculature of the neck. When the neck appears long and thin, this indicates the predominance of vata dosha. When the neck appears shorter and thicker, as if the head were close to the shoulders, this suggests the role of kapha dosha. Once again, pitta is more moderate, between the two.

The Hand

When observing the hand, you can observe both the fingers and the palm. The fingers reflect the same findings you saw in the bones. Those that are narrow and long suggest vata. Those that are shorter and thicker suggest kapha. Those that are in between suggest pitta. The shape of the palm will either be square or rectangular depending upon the length of the metacarpal bones (the bones in the hand). Long bones produce a rectangular shaped palm. Moderate and shorter bones produce a square palm. Thus, those with a predominantly vata constitution will more likely have a rectangular shaped palm. Those with a pitta and kapha constitution will more likely have a square palm. In order to tell the difference between the pitta palm and the kapha palm, it is necessary to look at the fleshiness of the palm. A thicker, meatier hand suggests more kapha.

Fingernails

The fingernails are generated primarily by the earth element and so we see that those with a kapha nature tend to have the strongest and thickest nails that are least likely to break. Those with a vata nature, being the most subtle and least dense of the three doshic types, have the thinnest and most fragile nails that break easily. Those with a pitta nature, being slightly denser by nature than vata and less so than kapha, have a thickness between the two.

Body Build, Weight and Musculature

The mass of the body is greatest in those with a predominantly kapha nature. This is because those with a kapha nature have a greater amount of the earth element in their structure and this brings dense and gross (larger and obvious) attributes to the body. As a result, there is a naturally greater amount of body fat and musculature creating a stocky nature. Those with a vata nature, having a predominance of the ether and air elements in their constitution, have the least body mass. This produces less musculature and body fat. As a result, the bones appear more prominent, especially around the shoulders. Those with a pitta nature, owing to a great amount of fire and a smaller amount of the water element, have a moderate body mass. The tissues produced have a higher metabolism which keeps them strong and lean. This has the potential to produce outstanding muscular definition. Body fat, though greater than in a person with a healthy vata nature, is still minimal.

A person's body build is the end result of the length and thickness of their bones and the amount of body fat and muscle that they maintain. Just as we compare the length of a bone to its circumference to determine doshic nature of the boney structure, we can do the same with the height of a person in relationship to the circumference measured around their chest, abdomen and thighs. Assessing body build can be achieved by a quick visual inspection and not by actually measuring body parts. Those with a kapha nature have an endomorphic body build (stocky). Those with a pitta nature have a mesomorphic body build (muscular) and those with a vata nature have an ectomorphic body build (lean and thin).

The Functions of Your Body

How your body functions tells a lot about your constitution, as well as any imbalances that are present. For instance, if you feel hot, there is more fire within you. If this has been true for most of your life and is not causing a problem, this is a constitutional tendency. It is likely that you have significant pitta in your nature. However, if this is a new phenomenon that has only recently occurred, you may have a pitta imbalance. Thus, it is only the long-term patterns that tell about your constitution, while short-term patterns tell about imbalances.

Appetite

Your appetite is a reflection of the dance between fire, air and water. Fire gives strength to the appetite as it seeks food to burn. Air feeds the fire but tends to blow irregularly. As a result, air makes the fire unstable and sometimes the appetite is strong and sometimes it is weak. Water protects against fire but it also tempers the fire and in doing so can lower the appetite.

Those of you with a pitta nature have a naturally strong digestive fire and this leads to a consistently strong appetite. A person with a predominantly pitta nature is not too picky about what or when they eat. If food is available and they have not eaten for a little while, their tendency is to eat the food. Those of you with a vata nature have a greater amount of air and this makes the fire unstable. As a result, the appetite tends to be more inconsistent and is easily disturbed. Circumstances and the environment must be just right or you may lose your appetite. Meanwhile, those of you with a kapha nature, owing to a greater amount of water in your constitution, have a consistently lower appetite. As a result, you become hungry less often and you are more likely to eat smaller amounts of food in one sitting. When you do eat, you are not too picky.

Digestion

The strong digestive fire in those of you with a pitta nature leads to strong digestion and relatively few symptoms of discomfort following a meal though, when symptoms do occur, they take the form of burning. The variable digestive fire of those with a vata nature leads to more frequent symptoms of digestive imbalance. There is a long-term tendency toward developing gas, bloating or cramping. The weak digestive fire found in those with a kapha nature leads to feelings of heaviness after eating. Food sits in the stomach and is digested slowly.

Elimination

The strong digestive fire in those of you with a pitta nature builds up more heat in the digestive system. This heat needs to be eliminated and, as a result, bowel movements are frequent and easy. A person with a pitta nature has 1-3 movements each day, rarely experiences constipation and may experience occasional loose stool. Those of you with a vata nature, having a variable fire, tend to have an irregular elimination pattern. This means that sometimes you may skip a day and sometimes you may have more than one movement in a day. Since the dry quality is also a part of the vata nature, the stools have a tendency to be drier and harder, and constipation is a fairly common challenge. Those with a kapha nature, having a weaker but steady digestive fire, tend to eliminate once per day and, owing to their moister nature, their stools tend to be softer and may occasionally have mucus in them.

Body Temperature

Body temperature is a function of the fire element. As a result, people with a pitta nature, having the greatest amount of fire in their constitution, tend to feel warm more often than others. They will be the first to kick off the covers on a warm night, first to put on the air conditioning and, even on a cool day, might wear shorts. Meanwhile, those with a vata nature tend to feel the coldest, owing to less fire in their nature along with a thinner body that does not retain heat. As a result, they are the first to put on an extra blanket at night, dislike air conditioning and, even on a somewhat warm day, might wear an extra layer or carry a shawl. Those with a kapha constitution have little fire in their nature as well. However, their body mass holds on to heat better than that of a person with a vata nature. As a result, body temperature is steadier and they do not easily become very cold or very warm.

Sweat

Sweat is a function of fire and water. When we are hot, our bodies sweat in an effort to reduce our body temperature. As water reaches the skin, evaporation cools the body. We sweat the most when we are well hydrated and hot. As a result, people with a pitta nature, having a predominance of fire and water in their constitution, tend to sweat the most. As fire has a sharp quality to it, it is natural for the sweat of a person with a pitta nature to have a sharper or stronger odor to it. Those with a kapha nature, having the greatest amount of water in their constitution, also tend to sweat easily. This is particularly true if they are exercising and building up the fire. However, their sweat will lack the strong, sharp quality and will smell more pleasant. Meanwhile, those with a vata nature, lacking in both fire and water, will not sweat very easily. Of course, even a person with a vata nature will sweat if they exercise to build up the fire and drink plenty of fluids.

Skin

The balance of the elements can be easily observed on the skin. Air makes the skin drier and rougher. Water makes the skin moister and smoother. Fire gives the skin luster and earth makes the skin thicker.

Those of you with a vata nature, having more air in your nature, and less fire, water and earth, will tend to have skin that is drier, rougher, thin and lacking in luster. Those of you with more pitta in your nature, having more fire and water, and less air and earth, will tend to have skin that is radiant and slightly moist or oily. The skin will have a moderate thickness, as some mass comes from water as well as earth. Those of you with a more kapha nature, owing to a greater amount of earth and water in your nature and less fire and air, will have skin that is thick, moist, soft and a little pale.

Menses

Menstrual flow and regularity are a function primarily of the water and fire elements. Water increases the quantity of the flow and fire increases the intensity of the flow. Air also plays an important role in that its dry quality reduces flow and its mobile quality disturbs the regularity of flow.

Those of you with a vata nature, having less water and fire and more air, tend to have an irregular flow with some menstrual periods being heavier and some lighter. In general, periods have a shorter and lighter flow lasting 1-3 days. In addition, the onset of flow is more inconsistent. For example, flow might occur one month after 22 days and another month after 35 days.

Those of you with more pitta in your constitution, having more fire and water and less air, tend to have more consistency in the onset of flow. Flow tends to be heavy for a few days then becomes spotty for a couple of more days. A typical menstrual period would last 3-5 days with three days of heavier flow.

Those of you with a more kapha nature, having the most water in your constitution and less fire and air, have the most consistent menstrual cycles and are mostly likely to sustain a 28-day cycle. The volume of flow is large, but it is not as intense as a person with a pitta nature. As a result, it lasts longer. A typical pattern is for a period to last 5-7 days with five days of heavier flow. In addition, there is a greater tendency toward having clumpy clots in the flow.

Sleep

Sleep is a function of the heavy qualities of earth and water. As a result, those with a kapha nature have the easiest time falling to sleep and staying asleep. It has been said that a person with a kapha nature could sleep through an earthquake. As a person with a vata constitution has the lightest nature, their sleep is easily disturbed by noises or their own thoughts and worries. It takes them longer to fall asleep and any disturbance can wake them up. Once awake, it can be difficult to go back to sleep. Those with a pitta nature sleep well in general and are only disturbed if it is too hot in the room. They may be awakened by noises at night but will fall back to sleep easily.

Exercise: Determine Your Constitution

Review the two charts below and circle the characteristics that apply to you. Since it can be difficult to perceive yourself accurately, you may wish to ask a friend for his / her thoughts as well. If you are still not sure of which description to circle for a particular characteristic, just leave it blank and go on to the next one. You do not need to circle a response for each characteristic in order to accurately determine your constitution. However, the more characteristics you include, the more accurate your final determination will be. One of the charts is for body structure and the other one is for body function.

When reviewing the body function chart, note your long-term tendencies and do not consider how your body has been functioning for the past few days or weeks. It is your long-term tendencies that are useful for determining your constitution.

When you are done, add up the columns and then combine the results of the two charts together. The combined results will give you the best indication of your constitution. These numbers represent an approximate ratio of the amounts of vata, pitta and kapha in your constitution.

Determining the Percentage of Vata, Pitta and Kapha in your Constitution

Body Structure	Vata	Pitta	Kapha
Face	Oblong or narrow	Angular with strong features	Round with soft features
Eyes	Small	Deep set, medium	Large
Nose Bridge	Narrow width to the bridge	Medium width to the bridge	Wider and fatter
Lips	Thin	Medium	Full
Complextion	Lack Luster or a dusty gray	Rosy, ruddy	Pale
Hair	Coarse fibers but scanty and dry	Fine fiber, oily, may experience early gray	Coarse fibers, oily, and quite full or dense
Skin	The skin is thin	The skin has a medium thickness	The skin is thick
Bones	The length to width ratio makes the bone appear narrow	The length to width ratio is moderate	The length to width ratio makes the bones stocky or stout
Neck	Long	Medium	Short
Hand	Rectangular palm with narrow fingers	Square palm and medium fingers	Square, fleshy palms with short or stout fingers
Fingernails	Thin and may be fragile	Medium and stronger	Thick and strongest
Weight/Bodyfat	Light or has frequent ups and downs	Moderate and relatively steady with a slow gain during the midlife years	Tends to be consistently heavy and stocky throughout life
Musculature	Minimal	Moderate, strong and reasonably well defined	Bulky, stocky
Body Build	Ectomorph	Mesomorph	Endomorph
Chart Totals			

Body Function	Vata	Pitta	Kapha
Appetite	Picky, variable, sometimes forgets to eat, and little things can cause you to loose your appetite.	Consistently strong and not easily lost.	Consistently low.
Digestion	Gas and bloating occur frequently. Gas has little odor.	Burning indigestion or smelly gas are common challenges.	Feels heavy after meals. Food does not seem to digest for a long time.
Elimination	Stools are hard. There is straining. Sometimes skips days.	Softer and sometimes loose. Elimination occurs 1-3 times per day.	Stools occur only once per day, they are almost always solid and log like. If out of balance, there may be mucous in the stool.
Sweat	Does not sweat easily.	Sweats easily and has stronger body odor.	Sweats easily with exercise. There is a pleasant body odor.
Body Temperature	Feels cold easily and enjoys the heat.	Often feels warm and enjoys cool temperatures.	Does not feel too warm or too cold too often.
Skin	Skin is dry and rough. Lips may crack.	Skin is oily with a tendency to develop red rashes or acne.	Skin is soft and moist. If problems develop, they are moist and oily.
Menses	The cycle is often irregular and painful. Bleeding is light and lasts 2-4 days.	The cycle is regular and the flow is heavy for 3-5 days.	The cycle is regular, flow is moderate and lasts 5-7 days.
Sleep	Sleep is light and easily disturbed. There may be frequent periods of insomnia.	Falls asleep easily and sleeps well most of the time unless it is too hot.	Falls asleep easily and sleeps deeply. Rarely wakes up from noises and may be hard to awaken.
Chart Totals			
Total (Structure and Function Combined)			

Personal Reflections

My Own Constitution

Take a look at my picture: what do you think my constitution is? Take a look at the shape of my face, my eyes, nose and lips. Look at my neck and my upper body to get a sense of my musculature and body tissue. What do you think? Here is a little bit more about my long-term tendencies: I have always had a good appetite and when I was less disciplined, after eating my own meal, I'd glance at my wife's plate to see what she had left behind. I was never shy to finish her meal. I was also never very picky. Through most of my adult life, I had 2-3 soft bowel movements per day. My sleep is also generally good, though it can take a little while to fall asleep and I wake up if there are noises. When I am stressed, my sleep is often disturbed. It can be both difficult to fall asleep and if I wake up, difficult to go back to sleep. Generally though, I go back to sleep quite easily. My skin is a little oily and, as a teen, I had acne that was quite intense. I sweat pretty easily but it does not have a strong odor unless I eat or drink pitta-aggravating foods such as coffee. (Red meat and alcohol also cause strong odor as, they too, aggravate pitta). When my diet isn't quite right, I get gas and it tends to have a strong odor. I don't generally feel warm or cool too easily. Do you know my constitution? You might want to wait till the end of the next section on psychology to learn a little more about me.

Keep your Evaluation in Perspective

Having evaluated thousands of patients over the years, many of whom have tried to evaluate themselves, I can say that any chart or table is only as accurate as your self perception. Our perception of ourselves is often inaccurate, as we tend to see ourselves more the way we want to be rather than the way we are. Sometimes, though, our self perceptions are skewed in the other direction and we may have a negative self image. Therefore, it is helpful to work on the chart with a friend. It is also more fun, and you can both look in the mirror and compare your features. However, some of the more nuanced determinations are still challenging, unless you have some experience looking at this sort of thing. For the most part, when one dosha is predominant, it is not difficult for the pattern to emerge and reveal the nature of a person. However, some people are more complicated and, for this reason, being evaluated by a trained ayurvedic health professional is helpful.

LESSON 6: CONSTITUTION, PERSONALITY AND THE MIND

*If the mind is like a monkey, moving about all
the time, your constitution determines where it goes.*

The Mind and the Constitution

Your mind has the same basic constitution as your body. The mind is considered a subtle body or an energetic template of the physical body. The same elements that mold the body at conception form the subtle body or mind. The Vedic idea of the mind is a bit different than the Western idea. The mind is understood to be the collective awareness of every cell in the body. It does not reside in the head but is experienced through the brain. The conscious mind represents only one aspect of our consciousness. Our subconscious, our deeper processes, are understood in Vedic thought to reside in the heart. While the mind processes truth, only the heart has the capacity to directly know truth. It is through the heart that we experience our divine connection. This is why words can never fully express a divine experience.

Just as your constitution reveals itself through the structure and function of your body, it also reveals itself through your personality. Just as everyone's body structure and function are different, so too is each person's personality. No two people were created alike. Even within each doshic type, there is a great range of possibilities. What we call the personality is a function of the balance of the three doshas, as well as a person's spiritual development. In other words, a person's personality is not fixed by the building blocks of nature. These elemental building blocks provide a strong structure for the personality but the energy that moves through that structure is the final determinant. As a person grows and evolves spiritually, the energy moving through the structure becomes purer and clearer. As that occurs, a person's personality becomes more fully established and that person becomes both self-confident and Self-confident. The Vedic term for this is "svastha". This term is used to describe perfect health and implies that, in order to attain perfect health, a person must become fully established in their true nature as spirit. As this occurs, the ego comes under control. With control over the ego comes control over behavior.

The mind is greatly affected by how we use the senses. Exposure to unhealthy sensory input is disturbing to the mind. Exposure to harmonious impressions through the senses brings calm and peace. It is the calm and peaceful mind that can realize its true nature as spirit, control the ego and bring behavior under control. The journey to create a calm and peaceful mind matches the journey to create perfect health. In other words, the path to enlightenment and the path to perfect health are one and the same. And thus, we see that Ayurveda and yoga are truly one science. They are like two sides of a coin, inseparable. Ayurveda provides the knowledge and tools to know how to live in a manner that will create optimal health. The practice of yoga provides the self-control necessary to succeed in living that life.

The Qualities of Nature and the Personality

As previously stated, the ten pairs of opposite qualities combine together to form the five elements. The five elements form the doshas and the balance of the doshas defines the constitution. The constitution can then be said to provide the basic shape of the body and mind. When understanding your personality, it is important to examine the qualities of your mind. From this understanding, the elemental and doshic balance are easier to see.

Qualities of Nature and their Effect on the Mind

Below is a listing of each quality in nature and several examples of how it can manifest in the mind. Note that the qualities can also combine together to create many effects.

Quality	Examples
Hot	Passion, intensity, understanding
Cold	Lacking in passion and intensity, aloof, distant
Heavy	Realistic, burdened, stubborn
Light	Unattached, unconcerned, fragile
Stable	Unwavering emotions, reliable, consistent, dependable, slow and steady
Mobile	Mood swings, impulsive, inconsistent
Moist	Empathetic, compassionate
Dry	Fragile, rigid, lacking in emotion
Sharp	Focused, direct
Dull	Impenetrable, difficulty taking in information, slow to respond
Cloudy	Difficulty understanding and perceiving things as they are
Clear	Very perceptible, able to take in more information
Hard	Rigid
Soft	Gentle
Gross	Realistic, practical
Subtle	Esoteric, inspired, creative
Dense	Slow to respond and understand
Flowing	Creative, expressive
Rough	Lacking in tact
Smooth	Tactful, gentle, kind

The Five Elements and the Qualities of the Mind

The ten pairs of opposite qualities combine together in forming the five elements. While these qualities can be observed in the mind, so too can the elements themselves. A person with lots of ether in their constitution has a more dreamy personality but might be called "spacey". One with more air has a quick wit but is also forgetful. Fire makes the mind crave information but can lead to arrogance. Water helps the mind develop compassion and empathy but also leads to attachment. Earth provides stability but also obstinance. Below is a more complete listing of how each element can be observed in the personality.

Qualities of the Elements and their Effects on the Mind

Element	Examples on How It Affects the Personality and the Mind
Ether	Esoteric, expansive, open minded, inspired, creative, dreamy, spacey
Air	Quick movement of thoughts, impulsive, takes initiative, forgetful
Fire	Digests information quickly, perception, discrimination, intensity
Water	Empathy, compassion, devotion, deep feelings, attachment
Earth	Stability, reliability, dependability, obstinance

The Three Doshas and the Mind

The five elements join together to form the three doshas, each dosha consisting of two main elements. These doshas are the forces that act on the mind. They are neither the qualities of nature nor the building blocks. They are the end product and the container of both. They play an important role in determining the types of thoughts and feelings that we experience. As you read through the personality descriptions below, remember that we are all a unique combination of the three doshas.

Vata Dosha and the Mind

If you have a vata nature, your mind will take on the qualities inherent in ether and air as they combine together. You will have a light mind. This means that you won't get too serious very often and if you do, it will pass quickly. You are generally enthusiastic and have a somewhat bubbly or vivacious personality. Your mind is mobile and moves quickly. This is reflected in your speech, which is fast and which rambles as the mind changes directions. As vata is subtle, your mind often goes into creative, inspired and esoteric realms. However, the subtle, light and mobile natures all combine together to make focusing more of a challenge. Thus, you may meander or drift from one interest to another. This can make finishing projects that once inspired you difficult. That same lack of focus can result in a tendency to misplace your belongings. Being light and mobile, you are open minded and not very attached. This can lead to inspiration but also impulsivity. Each new interest may seem like "it" to you and you will turn all of your energy toward that interest. However, when the next exciting interest arrives at your doorstep, you are likely to change direction once again. For instance, you might become very excited when meeting a spiritual teacher that you resonate with. However, this infatuation is short lived and when you find out about a new spiritual teacher, you won't hesitate to change teachers and turn all of their energy toward that teacher. This can occur again and again. The same process can occur in relationships, job interests and so on. Loyalty and steadfast devotion are not your natural virtues, though they can be cultivated through effort. Neither is sustainable passion. The cold nature of vata leads to a lack of passion about any one thing in life.

People with a vata nature like to explore many avenues.

The following scenario expresses the detached nature of a person with a vata nature and how that can lead to changing one's mind:

A woman with a vata nature is going to the movies with friends. A plan had been established to see a particular movie. When she arrives at the theater her two friends are arguing. One wants to change the movie they decided on because the review is not very good. The other wants to see the movie they set out to see just because that was the plan and it feels right to follow through. When she arrives, they both look to her and ask her what she wants to do. The person who wants to follow through explains why. The vata woman agrees and says, "Ok, let's go see the movie that we were going to see." But then the other person states her argument and explains that the reviews are very bad and that it won't be much fun. The vata woman again agrees and says, "Ok then, let's see another movie." The outcome of the argument does not matter much to the woman with a vata nature. She is neither greatly attached nor does she feel the need to persevere on finding the one "right" choice. What is really comes down to is that she just wants to have fun.

The same light quality that causes a person of vata nature to be less attached can also lead to mood swings. The combination of the light and mobile qualities can create instability in the mind. Just as an opinion might easily swing, so too can emotions. While you are enthusiastic and lighthearted by nature, your pendulum of balance does not stay in any one place for too long and can temporarily swing toward extremes when out of balance. Thus, happiness or unhappiness, irritability or joy, anxiety or confidence, each take their turn in the mind and neither pole generally stays for very long. These polar extremes can become more pronounced when a person of vata nature is under greater stress and severely out of balance.

Pitta Dosha and the Mind

If you have a pitta nature, your mind will take on the qualities of fire. Your mind will be hot, sharp and penetrating. This leads to greater focus and passion but also to taking life more seriously than others. When your mind becomes too hot and sharp, you will be prone to anger and intensity.

Of course, the fire in the mind also creates warmth and, as a result, you will be warm and friendly to those people that you like. However, if you do not like someone, you can be cruel toward them. Being sharp and focused, you can be very competitive. Your relationships may become divided in your mind between those you like and those you oppose. You are a formidable opponent.

Your mind is able to digest information rapidly and this leads you to quick conclusions, but a lack of patience with those who process information more slowly than you do. You will stand by your conclusions unless new information arrives. Information is the key to your mind. If new information contradicts your past conclusions, you won't hesitate to change your mind. So, while being convinced that you are right most of the time, you are not stubborn. You will change your opinion and even the direction of your entire life if new information makes it clear that that is the best choice. You are highly logical.

The sharpness of your personality causes your speech to be clear and to the point. You will speak emphatically with the presumption that you are right. This often appears arrogant to others but it is really an expression of your clear, precise and passionate nature. The pace of your speech is moderate and your words reflect the intellectual, analytical and logical nature of your mind. The combination of heat and light gives your voice passion as you illuminate your ideas. This charismatic quality makes you a very effective and believable speaker and helps you to win most arguments.

Focus is your strength. You have a good chance of accomplishing whatever you set out to do. You prefer to be organized, as this helps you to achieve your goals. When a challenge arrives, you are quick to formulate a plan and manage the problem. This can turn you into a productivity machine and you will need to be careful of workaholism and burnout.

The following example expresses the personality of a person of pitta nature with a sharp, clear mind:

Remember the story about the three people who meet at the theater to see a particular movie? One person read a review of the movie and saw that it was not very good, and was arguing that it did not make sense to follow through with the plan. This was the person with a pitta nature. She argued that it made sense to see a different movie with a better review. Let's continue the story. As the three people are discussing what movie to see, a couple walks by, overhears the conversation and stops. "Excuse me, we just saw the movie and we loved it. The review you read was completely wrong. I find that I often disagree with that particular movie critic. I think you will all like it very much. In fact, everyone I know liked the movie." Given that information, the person with the pitta nature acquiesces and decides that it is best to follow through with the original plan. Being right is important to the person with a pitta nature. However, what is right depends entirely on the information at hand. As information changes, so does the right choice.

While the sharp and clear qualities of your mind and your ability to quickly digest information leads you toward reasonable, logical conclusions, they can also lead to frustration when working closely with people who function differently. This is particularly true when you work with people who make decisions based on emotions or inspiration. It can be a challenge and a learning experience for you to accept the processes of others. Unless you are in balance, your frustration level will grow into anger.

Kapha Dosha and the Mind

If your constitution is mostly kapha, your mind will take on the qualities of water and earth. These elements, being heavy, cool, moist and stable, are reflected in a personality that is dependable and reliable. Emotions run deep but they are not easily expressed. Being cool and moist, the emotions that are most often felt are softer emotions, such as compassion, empathy and love. Lacking are the mood swings common to vata (air) and the passion and intensity common to pitta (fire).

Lacking in fire, your mind will work more slowly than that of a pitta. It will take time to metabolize information and integrate new concepts into your life. You like things the way they have been and the way they've already been planned. When you need to make a decision, you will take your time, consider all of the information, sleep on it if necessary and then come to a decision. Once you make that decision, you won't be easily swayed to change your mind. Others may perceive this as being stubborn, but it is really a reflection of the stable and heavy qualities of your nature.

Your speech reflects what is happening in your mind. You will speak slowly and deliberately. While you may not use many words, each one is well thought out and important. Your voice will be smooth, gentle, non threatening and melodious.

All in all, your gentle nature makes you well liked by others. Friendships and other relationships are important to you, and others appreciate your soft and dependable nature.

Remembering once again the story of the three friends who meet at the movie theater to see a movie, one person read a review of the movie and realizing that the movie was not supposed to be very good, argued to change the movie they were going to see. Another person held steady to their original plan in spite of the new information. The third person was easily convinced by both of them toward their own perspective and could, as a result, go either way. The person who held steady to the original plan and was uneasy about making a change was the person of kapha nature. Neither new information nor someone else's passion and inspiration are likely to motivate a person of kapha nature to make a sudden change.

Exercise: Determine your Psychological Constitution
- Below is a list of personality and mental characteristics for each doshic type. Circle the characteristics that apply to you the most. For many of the questions, it is best to consider how you are when you are under some stress and a little out of balance. Most of us are somewhat balanced between the three types when we are calm and in balance. A little stress reveals our tendencies and this is what you want to identify in the chart. If you are not sure of the answer to a question, consider asking someone who knows you. If you are still not clear, just omit that question. When determining your constitution, remember to look for long-term patterns (of how you react under stress) rather than occasional tendencies. Add up the columns

when you are done. See if your psychological nature matches your physical nature. They should be close. Next, you can add these numbers to the numbers you came up with from looking at your structure and function and then calculate the final percentages for your constitution. This method of determining constitution is highly reliable. However, ayurvedic practitioners also include pulse diagnosis into their evaluation and this brings in other important information.

Trait	Vata	Pitta	Kapha
Personality when balanced	Bubbly or enthusiastic	Focused and friendly	Kind and sweet
Roles in relationship to others	Cheers others on	Takes a leadership role	Prefers a quiet, supportive role
Mental Tendency under Stress	Becomes scattered or overwhelmed. Hard to deal with stress.	Becomes more intense, focused and develops a plan	Does not appear very affected by stress, may become quieter
Moods	Mood swings and anxiety are common	Becomes more critical and angry	Experiences melancholy
Decision Making	Often indecisive	Usually makes quick decisions and stays with them unless there is new information	Makes them slowly and sticks with them to the point of stubbornness
Voice and Speech	Fast speech with a tendency to ramble	Argumentative/convincing	Slow with few words
Projects Approach	Inspired to start but it can be difficult to finish	Inspired to begin and develops a clear plan to follow. Usually finishes what is begun. Likes efficiency.	Less inspired to start but once started will usually finish. Rarely in a rush.
Challenging Emotions	Nervousness, anxiety, worry and fluctuations of anxiety and depression	Anger, intensity, resentment, jealousy	Over-sentimentality, lethargy, uninspired, complacency or melancholy
Total			

Personal Reflections

My Constitution and My Personality

OK, here is a little more about me that you can use to determine my constitution. I can be very focused. I am also a warm and friendly person if I know you well. I am aloof and rather shy if I don't. I do not generally have lots of friends but the friendships I make are deep, important to me and last a long time. I can be very enthusiastic especially if I am comfortable. When I speak to groups, I am clear and organized but I also get naturally excited about what I love to talk about which is, of course, Ayurveda. I often take a leadership position, as I have with the California College of Ayurveda and our National and State Associations for which I am a founding director. When I am under stress,

I may momentarily feel overwhelmed but that doesn't last long. I go into "fix it" mode and begin to plan my next move. Although I am not very moody, I can be critical and a bit intense. Still, I don't get angry often. I also experience a small amount of anxiety and fear for what might be coming around the corner. I am rarely ever depressed. When I talk, my thoughts are clear and concise. I am quick to give my opinion if asked; before I was more disciplined I would give my opinion even if no one asked for it. I won't shy away from a clean, healthy debate but I won't engage in arguments. I find that to be a waste of time and energy. When decisions need to be made, I can process information quickly and come to a decision. I am not stubborn and I will change my mind if there is information I did not consider. Well, what do you think? See page 55 and read the personal reflections. You'll find out my constitution there.

What if your body and mind appear to have different constitutions?

This is not supposed to happen, so something is wrong. Either the determination was wrong or one of the two is really an imbalance. Any dosha can be out of balance and appear predominant in the body and/or mind for a while. See the next section for more about imbalances.

LESSON 7: KNOW THE NATURE OF YOUR IMBALANCES

*"Having a birth certificate is important, but
so is a driver's license with your current address."*

Knowing your constitution is only one important part of understanding how to live your life. By defining your starting point, it is useful for learning how to prevent disease. The other important part is to know the current state of the doshas within you and the nature of any imbalances. This knowledge is essential for healing. While a person's constitution is called their prakruti, a person's current state and imbalance is called vikruti.

While everyone has an inherent unique balance of the three doshas, known as their constitution, any dosha can become disturbed. A disturbance in a dosha is generally defined as that dosha increasing beyond its normal proportion relative to the other doshas. However, it is possible for two or even all three doshas to be simultaneously disturbed at the same time. The more a dosha increases, the greater the symptoms that dosha produces, and the more difficult it is to treat. When two or three doshas have moved out of balance, the condition is even more difficult. But, never give up hope because as long as healing is possible, Ayurveda can and will help you to return to balance and, in doing so, maximize your healing potential.

Recall that the qualities of nature make up the five elements and that the five elements are the building blocks of all aspects of creation. This includes the symptoms of disease. Thus, at the root of a symptom lie both an elemental disturbance and an excess of one or more qualities. This creates an increase in the influence of a dosha and disturbs the physiology of the body and mind. The result is disease.

To know the nature of a disease (symptom) is to know its qualities. In the West, sometimes we name a disease after the person who identified it. Or, sometimes we name a disease using a Greek- or Latin-root word that relates to the part of the body affected. Arthritis, for example, comes from the Latin root *arthra*, which means joint, and the suffix – itis, which means inflammation. However, to truly know disease requires knowing its qualities. Like the story of Rapunzel, knowing the true name of a symptom (its qualities) gives you great power over it. Only with this knowledge can you alter your lifestyle or use herbs in such a way as to counteract the disturbed quality and return the body to balance. As this occurs, the underlying cause of the condition is removed and the damaged tissue heals.

As an example, imagine a pain in your body. Ask yourself, what are its qualities? Perhaps it is hot (inflamed) and sharp. If so, applying ice is a better treatment than applying heat, as the ice pack counteracts the qualities of the condition. Internally, avoiding excessively hot and sharp qualities are also important. Many spices, such as hot peppers, are hot and sharp and should be avoided. Foods such as milk and rice are dull and cooling. These can be increased in the diet. Practitioners of Ayurveda take this a step further and prepare poultices that use cool, dull herbs and also prescribe similar herbs for internal use that work specifically on the part of the body affected.

Once we know the nature of our imbalances, it is not only important to restore the proper balance of qualities but also to examine our lifestyle and try to understand what led to the imbalance in the first place. There are many layers to the cause of disease. If we penetrate the cause deeply enough, when we get close to the core we discover that we participate in creating the disease. Through the process of self observation and reflection we can discover what our role is. This provides us with the opportunity to do something about it. Some aspect of our core self must change for complete healing to occur. This process of self-observation and reflection accelerates our personal growth. Each symptom is looked at in a new light. Rather than as a problem, it becomes our teacher. Each symptom is the body's voice trying to communicate that something in our life is out of harmony. If we can solve the mystery, important lessons are learned and we have the opportunity for true healing to take place.

Using the example of the hot, sharp pain of arthritis, there are several possible levels of cause and several possible levels of healing. Let's look at the levels of cause first. On one level, it could be caused by the regular use of hot, sharp substances such as hot peppers and alcohol. On a deeper level of lifestyle, it could be caused by an intense (hot and sharp) and pressure-filled lifestyle. On a psychological level, it could be caused by an excessively hot and sharp personality.

Healing can also take place on many levels. On the most superficial level, healing can take place through the use of cooling and dulling drugs or herbs. This requires no change on the part of the person and the condition feels better, at least for a while. Deeper healing means removing the cause. Since there are many possible layers of cause, each should be examined and then, if needed, addressed. Healing on a deeper level often means changing one's diet to exclude hot and sharp substances and include more cooling and dull substances. This lifestyle change is very powerful. It works more slowly than drugs but eventually the pain and discomfort is controlled and the condition is less likely to return. Healing may need to occur on a deeper level still and could involve changing one's approach to life. An intense lifestyle filled with pressure and deadlines has a hot and sharp quality. Making lifestyle changes to reduce the pressure and intensity reflects a high level of awareness and leads to deeper healing. The deepest level of healing occurs when the realization takes place that the condition is caused by an aspect of the personality. A hot and sharp personality is one that is highly critical, intense and often controlling. Healing at this level means altering one's self-expression. For this to be successful, it must be true and not forced. Thus, in this case it must come from the cultivation of non-judgment and compassion. When this change is made, there is an increase in calmness and coolness. The entire world around that person seems to change. Everything, including work, becomes less intense. Other people seem nicer and more cooperative. When a person practices and lives in a new and healthier manner, their life has truly been transformed. With that transformation, the deepest level of healing is achieved. This is the healing of consciousness. The deeper the level of the healing, the slower it occurs, but the more meaningful and important it is. This is the truth of ayurvedic healing.

Below is a chart of the ten pairs of opposite qualities with examples of symptoms that can be produced in the body and mind when they become excessive.

The 20 Qualities of Nature and Examples of Symptoms

Diseases can be understood as disturbances in the qualities of the body and of the three doshas. Let's look at symptoms of excesses of the 20 qualities of nature. Note that most symptoms are caused by a disturbance in more than one quality.

Quality	Examples
Hot	Fever, inflammation, red face, red eyes, red rashes, burning urination
Cold	Chills, goose bumps, cold hands
Moist	Swelling, mucous, wet cough
Dry	Dry skin, dry eyes, dry vagina, constipation
Heavy	Weight gain, sluggish digestion
Light	Weight loss, muscle atrophy, light headed
Mobile	Shifting pain, rambling speech, hyper-mobile joints, nervousness, anxiety
Stable	Melancholy, stubborn tendencies, frozen shoulder
Sharp	Sharp pain, being too critical, intense or focused
Dull	Dull pain, difficulty understanding concepts
Hard	Hard stools, hard tumors
Soft	Obesity, loose stools
Gross	Obesity, enlarged organs
Subtle	Weight loss, muscle atrophy, vague discomfort
Dense	Tumors, excessive muscular development
Flowing	Excessive or prolonged menstruation, inability to control urination or bowel movements

The Unfolding of Disease

When a dosha becomes imbalanced, there is an increase in the influence of the elements and the corresponding qualities that make up that dosha. Ayurveda teaches that imbalances follow a basic pattern of flow. Once we forget our true nature as spirit, we begin to act disharmoniously and get caught up in the dramas of everyday life. The first sign of disturbance in the body can be found in the digestive system. This can be very mild and may be hardly noticeable at all, except for a little gas, burning, constipation, loose stools or a feeling of heaviness. As the doshic disturbance becomes worse, the condition spreads from the digestive system into circulation. The excess dosha and qualities then begin to mingle with the tissues and organs of the body where they produce additional symptoms of mild disturbance. If there is a pre-existing weakness in a tissue or organ, that structure is more susceptible to the disturbed dosha and its qualities. The dosha may then settle into that tissue. There, the imbalance begins to grow and greater and greater symptoms are produced. The origin of the pre-existing tissue weakness may be genetic or it may be due to past illness that caused some damage to the tissue.

Thus, in addition to helping people to develop a healthy lifestyle, Ayurveda places great emphasis on making sure that the digestive system stays healthy, making sure that only the proper qualities are taken into the body. I will comment on this idea further during *Lesson 9: Healing your Life Through Diet*.

Symptoms Due to Vata

When the vata dosha becomes imbalanced, there is an increase in the influence of the air and ether elements. This, of course, leads to an increase in their qualities within the body and mind.

Symptoms may be noticeable early on in the digestive system. The dry and hard qualities of vata can be seen in the stools which become difficult to eliminate. As air increases, gas forms and distention takes place. As the imbalance spreads to the circulatory system, the body becomes drier and colder. There may be dry skin, dry eyes and dry lips. As a person become colder they become uncomfortable in cold weather and are easily chilled. These are mild symptoms until the conditions settles into a weakened area. There the symptoms become worse. Any of the symptoms noted thus far can become much worse if the dosha settles into that location. In addition, if the dosha settles into the muscles, there may be cramping pain, weakness and atrophy (loss of muscle). There may be weight loss. Bones become more brittle (osteoporosis) along with the nails. There may be spotty hair loss and thinning. The nervous system may become more sensitive and there may be tremors, tics and twitches. The reproductive system may become weaker resulting in defects in the sperm or egg, resulting in infertility. Menses may become spotty and irregular as well. Of course, rarely do all of these symptoms occur in a single person and some of these symptoms may take decades to develop - one important reason why early intervention is important.

The mind can also be affected by a vata dosha disturbance. When it becomes disturbed, dramas are imagined that create greater anxiety, worry and fear. These are not the symptoms that arise from a true threat, rather they arise when there is no true threat present or out of proportion when only a minor threat is present. When the vata dosha has settled into the mind, there are often feelings of confusion and overwhelm as attention becomes difficult to focus.

Symptoms Due to Pitta

When the pitta dosha becomes imbalanced, there is an increase in the influence of the fire and water elements. This, of course, leads to an increase in their qualities within the body and mind. Of the two elements, fire is predominant.

As heat builds up in the digestive system, the first symptoms to develop are often mild burning, or frequent and loose stools. Gas may also form but pitta gas differs from vata gas as it has a sharp, foul odor. As the imbalance spreads to the circulatory system, the body becomes warmer and some of the tissues of the body experience mild burning sensations. This is common in the eyes but also may present as burning urination, burning inside the nostrils and burning of the rectum during bowel movements. As a person becomes warmer, they become uncomfortable in hot weather and seek out cool or air-conditioned places. All of these are mild symptoms until the condition settles into a weakened area. There, the symptoms become worse. Any of the symptoms noted thus far can become much worse if the dosha settles into that location. Two of the most common advanced symptoms of pitta imbalance are inflammation and infection. This occurs in any tissue that the pitta dosha settles in. Inflammation is common in the muscles, tendons and ligaments and results in joint and body aches and pains. Infections anywhere in the body, especially when accompanied by a fever, are due to an imbalance in pitta. Examples include urinary system infections and hepatitis. If pitta settles into the skin, a person develops angry red rashes, such as hives or acne, and ulcerations may appear on the skin or lips, as occurs in herpes simplex infections. If the dosha settles into the nervous system there may be burning nerve sensations going down an arm, a leg or the side of the face. In the reproductive system, the heat can damage the eggs or the sperm. Menstrual bleeding tends to increase in intensity.

Once again, rarely do all of these symptoms occur in one person. The symptom(s) a person develops depends upon the tissues that have been previously weakened and are now susceptible.

The mind can also be affected by a pitta dosha imbalance. As the mind becomes disturbed, heated emotions become more dramatic. There is greater anger and intensity. The mind becomes more critical and cynical. The drive to be right and to win in a conflict or contest becomes more and more consuming.

Symptoms Due to Kapha
When the kapha dosha becomes imbalanced, there is an increase in the influence of the water and earth elements, leading to an increase in their qualities within the body and mind. Earth and water mix together and the imbalance has qualities similar to mud. Mucus formation is a primary symptom. Mucus is the mud of the body.

Symptoms may be noticeable early on in the digestive system. Moist heaviness reduces the strength of digestion and leads to a feeling of heaviness in the abdomen and a loss of appetite. The stools may become pale or covered with a thin film of mucus. As the imbalance spreads to the circulatory system, the body becomes more fluidic and sluggish. There may be generalized signs of water retention, such as slight swelling in the ankles and bloating around the abdomen. The eyes may produce more excretion and there may be a mild runny nose or post nasal drip. A mild lethargy and loss of motivation also begins. These are all mild symptoms and may or may not be noticeable until the condition settles into a weakened area. There the symptoms worsen. Any of the symptoms noted thus far can become much worse if the dosha settles into that location. If the dosha settles into the muscles, they become heavy and it feels like it takes more energy just to move the arms or legs. Tumor growth (mostly benign) can occur anywhere in the body, along with fluid filled cysts. The nervous system becomes sluggish and reflexes and reaction times slow down. Flow in the body of urine, stools, menses or blood slow down and can sometimes become obstructed by masses as they grow. An example of this is the obstruction of blood flow by deposits of cholesterol in the arteries.

The mind can also be affected by a kapha dosha disturbance. When it becomes disturbed, the mind slows down along with the ability to process information. There is loss of motivation and melancholy sets in.

Exercise

Below is a list of physical and emotional symptoms that are generally related to a specific dosha. As you read through the list of symptoms, circle any symptoms that are troubling you. You may see a pattern that shows which dosha is most out of balance with you. Of course, you can have imbalances in two or even three doshas.

Summary of Symptoms Related to Each Dosha

Vata	Pitta	Kapha
Gas and distention	Burning indigestion or occasional but strong smelling gas	Appetite loss and sluggish digestion
Constipation	Loose stools	Mucusy stools
Dry skin	Reddened rashes and acne	Feelings of heaviness in the abdomen
Cold sensitivity	Heat sensitivity	Water retention and swelling
Cramping, shooting, electrical or chronic pain	Burning or searing pains	Dull, achy pain
Weak bones (osteoporosis), joint pains or fragile nails	Red eyes	Excess eye excretions
Spotty hair loss	Inflammation anywhere in the body	Muscle heaviness
Tremors, tics and twitches	Infections anywhere in the body	Benign tumors and cysts
Infertility due to weakness of the egg or sperm	Anger, intensity or too critical	Difficulty processing information
Irregular and/or spotty menses	Sharper words	Lethargy
Anxiety, worry or overwhelm	Loss of patience, demanding	Melancholy, quieter than usual
Increased rambling in the voice		Not noticeable
Mood swings		

Personal Reflections

Most of my life, I tended toward pitta imbalances. As a teen, I suffered from some pretty intense acne. This is consistent with my constitution which is about 60% pitta, 20% vata and 20 % kapha. We all tend to go out of balance within our dominant dosha. However, any dosha can become disturbed and sometimes vata would go out of balance within me as well. I would often find myself anxious in social situations.

When I was crippled by what appeared to be an autoimmune disorder, my condition was caused by a vata-pitta combination of imbalances. This was consistent with the stresses and instabilities present in my life at that time. The vata part of the imbalance caused the joint pains to move around my body, weakened my joints, caused me to lose weight and made my nervous system highly sensitive. The pitta part resulted in excess heat that caused my joints to become red and inflamed. My eyes were very red too. My skin became sensitive to the sun and I ran a very high fever. Today, as I have learned to live more harmoniously, improved my lifestyle and learned to use my senses properly, I have only a mild vata or pitta imbalance from time to time and I rarely get sick. However, I am not impervious to imbalances. When my vata rises, I begin to lose things and my sleep will become disturbed. When my pitta rises, I find myself having less patience with others and my voice and actions become sharper.

LESSON 8: HEALING YOUR LIFE: THE PROCESS AND THE JOURNEY

*"Common sense: So easy to understand,
so difficult to practice."*

The process of healing has many layers, beginning with the alleviation of the most obvious symptoms all the way to attaining a state of existence where we fully express who we are physically and emotionally and reach our full potential as healthy human beings. Beyond this is the realm of the spirit. When our consciousness fully realizes our true nature as spirit, we not only experience perfect health, we are freed from worldly existence and merge like a drop of water back into the ocean of pure existence. This is the most important adventure of our lives. Restoring our body and mind to a state of perfect balance requires surrounding ourselves with an environment that takes into consideration our constitution and the nature of any imbalances that are present. Success on the journey requires great patience as well as persistence.

The path of healing through Ayurveda and yoga is a path of personal responsibility. Each person is empowered with the ability to make choices. Those choices will either bring health and peace of mind or suffering and disease. Most people make their choices about how to live based on a lack of knowledge. Taking cues from friends, family and the media, choices are made. If these choices have led you to optimal health and inner peace, then you have been blessed. But if not, Ayurveda outlines a clear road map for the journey and provides you with the knowledge and tools needed to succeed.

The path of healing is based on a simple premise. If there is an excess of a particular quality in your body or mind, then reducing your exposure to that quality and taking in the opposite quality will assist your body and mind in returning to its proper balance. It is really just common sense. By adjusting the qualities we take in, the elemental balance of the body is changed and with that, the physiological forces (doshas) that govern its function. As proper doshic balance is reestablished, normal physiology is restored and healing takes place.

The Balancing Qualities for Each Dosha

You are healed by the qualities that oppose those of the imbalance or disease. Below is a table of the qualities that help keep each dosha in balance. These are the qualities that lower or reduce the impact of the dosha.

Balancing Qualities	Vata	Pitta	Kapha
Warm/Cool	Warm	Cool	Warm
Heavy/Light	Heavy	Heavy	Light
Moist/Dry	Moist	Dry	Dry
Mobile/Stable	Stable	Stable	Mobile
Sharp/Dull	Dull	Dull	Sharp
Hard/Soft	Soft	Soft	Hard
Gross/Subtle	Gross	Gross	Subtle
Dense/Flowing	Dense	Dense	Flowing
Rough/Smooth	Smooth	Smooth	Rough
Cloudy/Clear	Cloudy	Cloudy	Clear

Exercise:

Let's see how much you understand. See how many of the following questions you answer correctly. I'll bet that if you made it this far through the book, you already have learned a lot and that you can figure out the answer to most of the following questions. The answers to the questions are below.

1. If a person had a fever, would it be a good idea to rest in the sun?
2. If a person feels cold easily, should they drink ice water?
3. If a person has an overactive mind, should they rest more?
4. If a person is depressed, might going for a run help?
5. If a person gets anxious easily, is it a good idea to go jogging on a regular basis?
6. If a person has a red hot rash on their body, is a warm shower a good idea?

1: No; 2: No; 3: Yes; 4: Yes; 5: No; 6: No

LESSON 9: HEALING YOUR LIFE THROUGH DIET

There are few things that are more important to our health and well-being than what we eat and how we digest our food. Healing our lives often means healing our relationship to food. The foods that we eat and how we eat them have a profound effect upon our well-being.

The Story of What Happened When Humans Disrespected the Plants

The following is a story that has been told to me by my teachers. It is a very old story with roots deep in the Vedic tradition. It is not meant to be taken has historical fact but rather as parable that teaches the wisdom of the Vedas. I have slightly adapted it for modern times.

Once upon a time, God placed the plants on the planet for the animals to consume. The purpose of the plants was to sustain animal life. Thus, they did not mind being consumed. In fact, by fulfilling their purpose in life, they continued their own evolution toward enlightenment.

For a long time, the plants and the humans lived in harmony. The plants thrived and the humans treated them with respect. Then, things began to change. The humans forgot that plants were life-forms worthy of respect and care. As a result, they began to abuse the plants. They no longer gave thanks to the plants for sustaining them. They began to consume more than they needed and they began to process the foods, changing their character and quality. All of this upset the plants. Not knowing what else to do, they went back to God. "God," they said, "we do not mind being consumed by the humans, this is our purpose. But the humans disrespect and abuse us and this is not right. What should we do?" God thought for a moment and pondered the situation. Then, he said, "If the humans disrespect you, then instead of the humans consuming you, you will consume the humans."

From that day onward, when the humans disrespected the food, the food caused the humans to get sick. This begins with indigestion. From an ayurvedic perspective, this is the start of the disease process. From the digestive system, the disease spreads to other parts of the body. Some of these diseases come on quickly while others take a longer time to develop. The wise individual, becoming conscious of this process, strives to heal his or her relationship with food. In doing so, digestion, health and well-being are improved.

Today, it is well understood that the choices we make regarding the quality and quantity of the food we consume is closely linked to many diseases. As a result, the traditional health community has joined the alternative health community in making some basic recommendations. These recommendations, if followed, will take the average person a giant leap closer to their health goals. Below are three basic guidelines that everyone agrees upon.

Consume Whole Foods that are not Processed

The foods we take should be fresh and less processed. The processing of food is well known to devitalize the food (destroying natural enzymes) and deplete important vitamins, minerals and trace nutrients (trace minerals, fiber, co-enzymes and much more). In recognition of this, the food industry sometimes replaces a token amount of the lost vitamins by adding synthetic versions. Not only are the minerals and trace nutrients not replaced in the processed food, the synthetic vitamins that are added back are poorly absorbed from the digestive system. This leaves the body deficient of many nutrients even though we feel full.

There is more damage done to the food than just the loss of nutrients. Through food processing, synthetic chemicals (food additives) are added to food to make it tastier, last longer and look prettier. These additives have no nutrient value. They are added to make foods thicker and creamier, more colorful, sweeter and so on. Some of these substances are already known to have deleterious effects. With many others, the long-term effect of consumption is not known. Every year, some chemical additives and processed ingredients (e.g. trans-fats) are banned from foods as their harmful effects become known. However, prior to their removal from store shelves, large amounts have been ingested by most people, often for decades.

Two supposedly natural (neither exists in nature in the form we consume it) but processed substances that are added to many foods and drinks are white sugar (sugar) and corn syrup (another sugary sweetener). Excesses of these substances in soft drinks and many other foods have contributed to the great challenge of obesity and its many complications, such as diabetes and heart disease. Sugar is so intensely pleasurable, and such an effective mood elevator, that we live in a society emotionally addicted to its consumption. Of all chemical addictions, society's addiction to sugar rules supreme affecting almost every adult and child in the United States, and leading to billions of dollars in health care costs due to related illnesses each year.

Ayurveda has long understood the concept of food processing. The ancient teachers wrote that the processing of food changed its qualities and usefulness. This is not always a bad thing. Some foods can become more digestible when processed. Cooking is the most common form of processing food. Other common forms include soaking beans and adding spices into the cooking process. While ancient ways focused on processing food to make it more digestible, modern technology has taken the concept in a different direction with a focus on preservation, increasing taste and improving consistency. Unfortunately, the end result has been to make the food less digestible. From an ayurvedic perspective, the heavy quality of food has increased. So too have the dull and soft qualities. These qualities increase the kapha dosha. As a result, many signs of imbalance can be observed such as obesity, diabetes and coronary artery disease.

Avoid Foods with Pesticides

Given a choice, how many consumers do you think would go into a restaurant and order a side dish of pesticide with their meal? Obviously no one would, and yet that is what happens every day. It not only happens at restaurants but in almost every home. Pesticides are in our children's breakfasts, lunches and dinners and even in the water. The toxic health challenges of these chemicals are well documented, yet economic concerns and lobbying by the pesticide and food industry have prevented their removal from all foods. What can you do? Shop at your local health food store or Co-op and buy organic. It may cost a little more but isn't your health worth the extra expense? Want to save money to make up the difference? Go out for one or two fewer meals each month or buy fewer coffee drinks in cafés. It's a matter of priorities.

Eat Less

Two simple words, and yet to follow them is among the most difficult tasks many people face. Self-control is a great challenge but if a person can be successful here, studies show that life can and will be extended. On the average, people consume 30% more food than they need. That adds up to a lot of extra pounds. Ayurvedic and yogic food guidelines have promoted for thousands of years the idea that a person should only eat till they are 75% full. The ancient yogic texts state that after a meal the stomach should be 50% full of food and 25% full of water. The remaining 25% should remain empty.

Ayurveda has taught the same basic principle and has explained that when too much food is consumed, even a healthy food becomes harmful. Any food taken in excess increases the heavy quality. This suppresses digestion beginning a cascade of events that lead to disease.

Most people have challenges with digestion. Whether it is gas, bloating, constipation, diarrhea, irritable bowel syndrome (IBS), hyperacidity or ulcers, digestive problems affect almost everyone. This is particularly significant as proper digestion is considered to be one of the three pillars that sustain life, the other two being proper rest and the proper management of sexual energy. When digestion is compromised the rest of the body will soon begin to suffer.

Healing the digestive system and managing our relationship with food are closely related. In order to heal our digestive systems, we must consider three areas: The first is how we eat. The second is what we eat. The third is how we combine our foods together. If we consume food properly, eat the proper foods and combine them together properly, I can confidently say that there is a 99% chance that your digestive challenges will heal themselves.

Challenges with Diet in the Modern Day

So many of the health challenges people face today are of their own making. Through the consumption of unhealthy junk foods, over-consumption and a general lack of awareness of how to properly consume food, we, as a society, have created a host of health challenges.

Many diseases have a strong relationship to an unhealthy diet. Obesity, high blood pressure, cardiovascular disease and diabetes mellitus are just a few examples. Cardiovascular disease (heart attacks and strokes) are the number one cause of death and are responsible for lowering the life expectancy by seven years! In fact, if a person has had one heart attack, life expectancy drops by 11.5 years.* Other diseases with known dietary components to their origin include many cancers, dementia, depression and arthritis. Many experts believe that diet and nutrition play a role in every disease! For all of the attention that the media has focused on diet, little has been accomplished. In fact, the rate of both childhood and adult obesity is rising. Clearly, what we, as a society, have been focusing on has not been working.

*American Heart Association Heart and Stroke Statistical Update, as published in Science Daily, January 2000

It is More Important How You Eat Than What You Eat

So much attention has been focused on the fad diet of the day. These diets generally make one recommendation that all people should follow and then focus almost entirely on what you eat rather than how you eat. None of them have been found to work on a consistent basis.

Ayurveda teaches that it is more important how you eat than what you eat. I often shock the students at the California College of Ayurveda when I tell them that I would rather see them eat a fast food hamburger properly than healthy foods like rice and vegetables improperly. Now, this is a bold statement, but hopefully it makes the point [and by the time you finish reading this section I hope you will agree].

Why is it so important how you eat? Because, no matter what you eat, if you don't digest it well you will not benefit from the food. Worse yet, Ayurveda teaches that the process of indigestion causes toxins (called ama) to form in the digestive system which spread to the tissues of your body. What exactly is ama? No one can say for sure. The ancient teachers of Ayurveda described it as having heavy, soft and moist qualities. The accumulation of ama has been said to lead to obstructions in the passages of the body. It interferes with circulation, elimination and cellular function. As the ancient teachers defined it only in general as "toxins", it is likely that ama is not one thing, but many. Ama is all of the unhealthy by-products and metabolites of poor digestion and is a contributing factor to most disease. Ayurveda focuses extensively on the prevention of ama formation through optimizing digestion. Once ama is present, Ayurveda focuses on the removal of ama through the proper application of purification techniques.

If you are curious about the amount of ama in your body, a clue can be found on your tongue. A normal tongue is pink and has no coating. Take a look in the mirror. If your tongue is coated with a brown, gray, yellow, green or white coating, ama is present. Ama also contributes to stronger body odor.

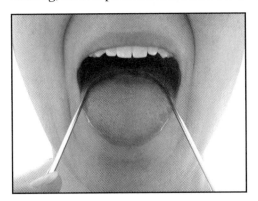

Conscious Eating and the Sacred

Eating is a sacred experience. After all, when you eat you are taking in atoms and molecules that are going to become a part of your body! These atoms and molecules have been around since the beginning of time. They originated in the comets and stars, float through space and enter our environment. They are constantly changing form and sometimes they make up the trees and plants and other times people and animals. When we take in food, we ask those same atoms and molecules to become a part of our bodies. In doing so, we are connecting to everything that has ever been, everything that is and everything that ever will be. When we eat consciously, we realize our connection to the greater whole and the interconnectedness of all existence. There is very little that is more sacred than this. Realizing this we form a very special and respectful connection to the food we are consuming.

Conscious Eating and the Ten Ayurvedic Guidelines to Assure Proper Digestion

To avoid the accumulation of ama in the body food must be digested well. There are ten general guidelines that, if followed, will help you to digest your food well. In doing so most of the symptoms of poor digestion such as gas, bloating, burning and heaviness after eating will disappear. So too will the coating on your tongue. The benefits extend to the mind as well and following these ten guidelines leads to greater feelings of calm and peace. And, if you are trying to lose weight, regardless of what you eat, if you follow these guidelines, you will be successful. The guidelines are:

1. Take Food in a Peaceful and Beautiful Environment.
Take a look at the environment that you eat your food in. Is it a calm and

peaceful place? Often it is not. Many people eat on the run, sometimes not even taking the time to sit down, much less care about the environment. Oftentimes, people eat in cluttered dining areas, noisy cafeterias under bright fluorescent lights, in the car on the way to work, or while engaged in conflict or debate. These environments make it nearly impossible to focus on the foods we are eating and how our body feels as it receives the food. When the environment is cluttered or active, the mind becomes cluttered and active making it difficult to focus. Agitation and distraction make it very difficult to control your eating habits.

If we consider that the environment where we are eating is Sacred, what can we do to sanctify it? Consider what type of music you are listening to while dining. Does it support a calm presence or is it distracting? What are you looking at while you eat? Are you watching television, reading or looking at a computer screen? Ask youself, "is this supporting being calm and peaceful?" Try the exercise below and see if you can honor the sacred while eating?

Exercise
- At home: Before eating, make sure that the eating area is clean and neat. Remove all papers and clutter. Consider the dining area to be sacred space. How is a church or temple taken care of? Keep it beautiful. Add flowers, plants and a candle to the space. Lighting a candle when you eat symbolizes the strength of your digestion. Turn off the television, it is too distracting. Would you have the television on in church? If you have music on, keep it beautiful and keep it in the background. If you live in nature, try keeping the music off and let nature be your personal orchestra.

- At work: If you can't find a quiet, peaceful and beautiful place to eat at work, consider bringing your lunch with you to a nearby park. If you go out to eat, consider the environment of the restaurant and chose a peaceful, quiet place.

2. Say Grace before Meals.
Sometimes, when a person thinks about saying grace before meals, an association is made to some past negative experience while growing up, or an association is made to a religious ritual. Either is often enough to put aside grace and just get to the food. Ayurveda and yoga offer another way of looking at grace.

Imagine that grace is just a moment in time where you can privately connect with the food and with all of the people who participated in helping your food get to your table. This grace honors and respects the food, the person who prepared your meal, and all of the hands, from the farmer to the people at the grocery store. Don't they all deserve some gratitude?

In Ayurveda, grace is not about God. It is about you and your connection to the Divine. It is a time to open your heart to those who helped to prepare the food and to prepare your body, mind and consciousness to receive the food. Grace opens the door into the temple and turns eating into a sacred experience. The calm created by saying grace focuses and prepares the digestive system so that when it receives the food, it can digest it properly preventing the formation of toxins.

Grace does not have to be religious, but it is spiritual. Going beyond the physical realm, grace helps us to connect to a larger picture of interconnectedness. We are all a part of an interconnected web of cooperative existence. Unless you are hunting, raising and growing all of your own food, you depend on a lot of people to get that food to your refrigerator. And, then there is the food itself and the intelligence that holds those atoms and molecules together. Through the food, you are connected to the process of creation itself. Most of those atoms and subatomic particles were formed within the stars and now will join your body. Like nothing else, the molecular transformation of the human body is a reminder of process of creation and destruction and the transience of life itself. When we eat, we are connecting ourselves to everything that has ever been and everything that will ever be.

Grace is a meditation that transforms eating from an ordinary experience to an extraordinary one. Grace opens the door to the sacred temple of the Divine. The Divine can take whatever form is dear to you. Whether it is Jesus Christ, Great Spirit, Nature, Krishna, Buddha, Allah or The Great Mystery, connecting with that which is greater than yourself is a humbling, harmonious, and healing experience.

Grace is a ceremony that honors your connection to the process. It is a ritual to call the attention of your consciousness to the present moment. Grace does not have to have a standardized form. Like spirituality, it can take whatever form is meaningful for you. As long as, through the process, you become conscious of the moment.

Grace-Filled Exercises

Create Your Own Grace: When creating your own grace, begin with asking yourself what is important to you about eating. Sit quietly and reflect from the heart on what you are thankful for? Grace can be said out loud or to yourself so no one needs to know what you say. If that is uncomfortable then simply enjoy a moment of silence and awareness of your own breath. In that moment be present with the experience of beginning a meal.

Use a Traditional Grace: A traditional grace is wonderful if the words that you say to yourself are heartfelt. Grace should never be about going through the motions because you feel you "should" do it. Each grace is a heartfelt experience.

A Simple Grace: This is a grace I often say. If you find it meaningful, you are welcome to share it. "Thank you, Great Spirit and Mother Earth, for this food I am about to eat. May it nourish me and give me strength so that I can be of service to others. Bless all of the hands that brought it to this table. And thank you to the food itself." I often end grace with "Om Shanti, Amen" which combines elements of my traditional heritage and my connection to yoga. The words Om Shanti mean "in peace."

Saying Grace in Public: It is natural to be somewhat self-conscious around others when saying grace. Usually, I say grace while bringing my hands together in prayer position. However, when I am in the company of those who do not know me very well, I may just lay my hands in my lap, close my eyes and say my grace. The times I have been "caught" in public while saying grace has always elicited respectful comments and never has anyone expressed offense. Even when eating at the table during a casual meeting, I will often say something like, "Pardon me, I like to take a moment of silence before I eat". This too has always been met with respect.

Saying Grace as a Family: It is a healthy and harmonious event when the family sits down together for a meal. In our home, we join together for dinner and sometimes for breakfast as well. I know that some people's family lives are crazier than our own. Saying grace together brings shared calm and sense of the sacred to the table. We often go around the table on different nights allowing each person to lead grace. Even when the kids get silly and say, "Rub a dub dub, thanks for the grub, yea God!" they are still participating, and a healthy habit is being created.

3. Eat Quietly and Avoid Conversations and Distracting Entertainment.
When you eat in silence, your mind is quieter and it is easier to be in a harmonious relationship with the food and your digestion will be improved. When we engage in conversation, read or watch television we miss important signals from our body and then we overeat. It's also difficult to chew food properly when we are distracted.

Exercises, Comments, and Suggestions
a) **Eat one meal alone and in silence:** Try eating one meal in complete silence with no distractions. It is easiest to do this the first time while eating alone. Avoid bringing a book or other forms of entertainment. If you are not at home, and you are uncomfortable being seen alone, go to a quiet, private place where you are less likely to be seen or known. A park is a good place. When all else fails, even a parked car on a hillside with a view will do just fine. Just avoid turning on the radio. After eating your first meal in silence, try it again another day. Over time, you will find yourself drawn to do this more often and you will become more comfortable with the silence and with being alone.

b) **Eating with family and close friends:** Explain that you are practicing conscious eating and are trying to eat in a calm and peaceful manner without great distractions. Don't expect others to be silent, but request that they not engage you in debate or controversy while eating. Try to keep the conversation about the food. Comment on the preparation and taste of the food. Keep all conversation light hearted. Since the dinner table is often a place where families work out problems or coordinate activities, suggest that you have a family meeting after dinner with some tea. If conversation does arise, and it often will, suggest that only positive conversing take place. Avoid all conflict and drama. It is always best to discuss the rules of the table with the family, and come to an agreement before coming to the table. If you have children at the table who get very noisy or silly, try creating an agreement where everybody takes five minutes of silence at the start of the meal. After five minutes, the energy will be much calmer. Any time the noise level rises too high you can take another five minutes.

c) **Eating with co-workers and others who are not engaged in conscious eating:** If you find yourself eating with other people who are not eating in a conscious manner, it is best to be the quieter one at the table. Rather than engage others in conversation, just sit back and relax. If you are drawn into a conversation, try giving a short but polite response.

4. Chew your Food Well.

If you are conscious (calm, quiet and present) while you eat your food, you will be able to chew your food well. Digestion of food begins with proper chewing. Chewing breaks down the food into small pieces and begins to separate the fiber (indigestible food matter) from the nutrient portion. Chewing food well also increases its surface area of the food allowing enzymes to work more effectively as they convert the food into small molecules that can be absorbed.

If you don't chew your food well, the rest of the digestive process will be compromised. Some disciplines recommend counting the number of times that you chew your food. Ayurveda teaches that the number is not important. What is important is that the food be an even, porridge-like consistency before swallowing. To achieve this you have to be present and that means avoiding distractions.

5. Take Food and Drinks Warm or at Room Temperature.

In general, warm food is digested better than cold food. Digestion itself is a process of cooking food. The strength of digestion is likened in Ayurveda to a fire. The fire transforms the food into the molecular nutrients that you will use to build new tissues.

When food is taken raw or cold from the refrigerator, it is harder to digest. How well you digest cold food will depend upon the strength of your own digestive fire (the power of digestion, ability to produce enzymes). For some people it is not a problem, but for many who experience excessive gas and bloating, this can make a very big difference. Taking food warm assists the body's natural digestive process. If you think of your digestion as a campfire, it is important to keep the fire healthy so that you can burn the food you put into it. A healthy fire transforms the food you put into it into nutrients. Since a fire is hot, anything cold antidotes its strength. Cooked and warm food support digestion. Food and drinks taken cold out of the refrigerator decreases it. As a rule, food and drinks are best taken at room temperature or warm, but never cold. Next time you drink water with a meal, hold the ice.

6. Food Should be Moist or a Little Oily.

In general, moist foods and those with a little oil are digested better than those that are too dry. The ayurvedic explanation is understandable. Dry food causes dryness of the mucous membranes of the digestive tract. The cells within the mucous membrane of the small intestine secrete many of the enzymes that help to digest the food. If the tissue is too dry, the secretion of digestive enzymes is diminished. In addition, dry foods lead to dry, hard stools and this makes constipation more likely. As elimination slows down, it is often more difficult to eliminate any gas that forms leading to bloating. So, feel good about adding a little oil to your meals but don't take too much.

7. Drink Only a Small Amount of Liquid with your Food.

Water and other fluids help to moisten the food and, as stated previously, are very beneficial. But, too much can be just as problematic as too little. If you take too much, you can alter the pH of the stomach acids and dilute the digestive enzymes and again interfere with their effectiveness. This is likened to putting water on a fire. If you put on too much, you will make it weaker.

How much is the right amount? In general, take ½ cup of room temperature liquid with each meal. Of course, if your meal is soup, you don't need to take much, if any, fluid. If you are taking something very dry, you may need a little more. Remember that a cup is 8 oz. and not the common 12 oz. mugs found in many homes and cafés. And it is most certainly not the 16 oz. Grande or 20 oz.Venti cups served at popular coffee houses. Size matters!

8. Eat until you are 75% full.

As stated above, this is one of the most important, and yet challenging, of the food guidelines for a majority of people. If you eat too much, even a good food can become toxic. Excessive food smothers the digestive fire, leading to poor digestion, a heavy feeling in the abdomen and lethargy after eating. Large meals overwhelm the ability of the body to produce digestive enzymes. The end result is the formation of ama and an increase in the kapha dosha. This is just as true for rice and vegetables as it is for pizza and hamburgers.

What does it mean to be 75% full? When the proper amount of food has been consumed, you will feel neither hungry nor heavy. A person who has consumed the proper amount of food feels "satisfied." The body feels light and the mind is clear.

The typical American idea of a good meal leaves a person feeling at least 100% full at its completion. While leaving a person with a satisfied feeling, there is also heaviness and lethargy following the meal. Most people do not realize that these are early symptoms of disease. Symptoms are the body's voice letting us know something is wrong. Feelings of heaviness and lethargy after a meal are communicating that you have eaten too much food. True, the body will eventually digest the food but through the process, the kapha dosha increases and ama is formed. This leads to weight gain and, if not managed properly, more serious diseases such as hypertension, diabetes and heart disease. Sometimes, the cause of a disease is as simple as eating too much on a habitual basis.

Most people are not conscious of the difference between feeling full and feeling satisfied. Due to eating while distracted, the subtle communication of the body to the mind is interfered with. The mind does not perceive that the body is satisfied. Distracted from the subtle calls of the body, a louder signal is required. Only when the stomach stretches in an unhealthy manner do most people become aware that they have had enough.

Exercise

Keep a food journal, and in that journal, write down the times that you eat each meal. After the meal, make a notation of how full you are. At first, it is difficult to judge, as there is little to compare how you feel to. Make a guess anyway. Each time you write down to what percent you are full, you will gain greater awareness of how you feel. This process helps you to become conscious. After a few days of becoming aware, try to become conscious as you are eating of when you get to 75%. And then stop.

9. Take Time to Rest After Meals.

If you are like many people, after your meal is done, you are ready to get on to the next activity. This is particularly true for people with a more pitta (focused and directed) nature. To the determined pitta, resting is an uncomfortable waste of time. There are plans to make and things to do. Often the mind has wandered on to the next activity as soon as, or even just before, the last bite is taken.

It takes the body several hours to fully digest a meal. In the stomach, hydrochloric acid and pepsin act on the food as the stomach churns the food into a mushy mass. That mass passes into the small intestine where enzymes continue the digestive process, converting the proteins, fats and carbohydrates into their molecular building blocks. These, along with additional vitamins and minerals in the food and water, are then absorbed. In the large intestine, more water is absorbed and the indigestible and non-absorbable remains are formed into fecal matter.

The more you can rest after a meal, the better for your digestion. Activity causes the physiology of your body to shift away from digestion and toward action. When you become active, the small blood vessels in the digestive system through which nutrients are absorbed constrict. This decreases absorption. Meanwhile, the blood vessels that bring blood to the muscles of your body dilate to allow them to receive more oxygen and nutrients. This situation worsens as soon as you encounter stress. The body treats stress just like exercise. It causes the small vessels of the digestive system to constrict, reducing nutrient absorption. Thus, going back to work or onto another activity right after eating, contributes to poor nutrient absorption. Stress also interferes with the secretion of digestive enzymes, decreasing the body's ability to digest the food properly in the first place.

Some people are given or take a lunch hour. Sadly, for many, that lunch hour has shrunk to 15-30 minutes. It is just not possible to eat a meal and then digest it well if all you have is 15 minutes and then hurry back to work. However, it does not take as much time as you might think. If you are eating your food consciously in a peaceful environment, it only takes about 15-20 minutes to eat a meal. It generally takes people longer than this to eat because they are engaged in debate, discussion or distraction. Following eating, take 15-20 minutes to rest. This is a good time for light conversation, a slow walk, light reading or to just gaze off into the distance and reflect. If you do find yourself pressed for time, try just taking enough time to close your eyes and take 3 conscious slow breaths. This will help close the door on the sacred experience of eating and keep you more relaxed as you re-enter your day.

10. Allow Three Hours or More between Meals.
It is important to allow food to digest and true hunger to return before taking another meal. Ayurveda teaches that taking food before true hunger returns leads to poor digestion. Using the analogy of a campfire, when wood is put onto the fire, at first it decreases the strength of the fire. Eventually, as the wood burns, the fire becomes stronger. At some time, it peaks. After that, it begins to die down, as there is not enough wood to sustain the fire. In the body, when there is not enough food to sustain the digestive fire, the fire calls out for more food. This is the appetite returning.

The body's digestive fire never actually goes out. If there is not enough food available, it will begin to slowly burn the tissues of the body. The body keeps a short supply of glucose (sugar for the blood) in storage. When that is used up, the body begins to burn stored fat. Later it burns up muscle and other proteins, until there is not enough structure to sustain life. This is what occurs during starvation. It occurs to a lesser extent during structured fasting and any time the gap between meals is too long.

When food is taken too soon after a previous meal, when the fire has not had time to complete the digestion of the previous meal, the digestive fire becomes weaker and it becomes hard to properly digest either meal. The effect is much like overeating and kapha is increased and toxins are produced. There is heaviness, bloating and lethargy.

Each meal should be taken when the previous meal has been digested, the body feels light and the true appetite has returned. Many people equate appetite with a sensory desire for more food. But this is not always the same. People often eat for emotional reasons, out of boredom or just for entertainment. This is considered a misuse of the sense of taste and it compromises your health. It takes a while to learn the difference between the desire for pleasure through food and true appetite.

Waiting at least three hours between meals is a good general guideline. This includes snacks. But, three hours is not a magic number. The ideal amount of time between meals depends upon the constitution and the nature of any imbalances present. Those with a kapha nature or imbalance should wait much longer.

People with a kapha nature, having a naturally slower digestive system, benefit by taking only two meals each day. Meal times at 10:00 am and 6:00 pm work very well. This helps to keep kapha dosha from further increasing and returns it to normal. While to some this may not seem often enough, remember that with a kapha imbalance there are already feelings of heaviness and lethargy and the weight of the body is above normal. Individuals with a kapha nature have a naturally low fire in their digestive system. By taking only two modest meals per day, not only will body weight return to normal but a person with a kapha nature will feel lighter and their mind will be clearer.

People with a pitta nature benefit most by taking three good meals each day. This can easily allow for five hours between meals. Meals can be taken at 7:30 am, 12:30 pm and 6:00 pm. These meals should be substantial, as pitta has a strong natural fire that digests the foods. If the three meals are substantial, there will be no hunger until the next meal and snacking will be avoided. Still, care should be taken to make sure that you have only reached the 75% full limit. It does take more food for a person of pitta nature to reach this level than a person of kapha or vata nature. For a person of pitta nature, the largest meal should be the mid-day meal as this is the time when Ayurveda teaches that the digestive fire is the strongest.

For a person of vata nature, it is important to take food more often than for a person of pitta or kapha nature. Taking meals every three hours is essential. Hypoglycemia (low blood sugar) is a common challenge for individuals with a vata nature or imbalance and, unfortunately, it is also more common for people with a vata nature or imbalance to skip meals or eat irregularly. The combination of hypoglycemic tendencies and a tendency to skip meals leads to low blood sugar and this produces greater anxiety, overwhelm and irritability.

Five meals per day is a good goal for a person with a vata constitution. However, these meals should not be very large. The strength of the digestive fire in a person with a vata nature or imbalance is not very strong and eating larger amounts of foods will lead to excessive gas and bloating. Thus, five small to moderate meals are most beneficial. A person who is trying to balance the vata dosha should take meals at 7:00 am, 10:00 am, 1:00 pm, 4:00 pm and 7:00 pm.

How Often Should You Eat?

Vata	Pitta	Kapha
5 times per day	3 times per day	2 times per day

It's Also Important What You Eat

Foods, like all of nature, are made up of the five elements and consist of a unique combination of the ten pairs of opposite qualities. By understanding the qualities inherent in a food and knowing the qualities inherent in a person, how the food and a person interact becomes known. No one food is perfectly healthy for everyone. Each person is unique and so too are the foods that will support them to thrive.

First and foremost, the foods that you eat should have the opposite qualities of any imbalance that might be present within you. If there is no significant imbalance, then the foods that are best are those with the opposite qualities of your constitution. Remember, if you tend to be cold, eating warm foods is best. If you tend to be heavy, it is best to eat light foods. If you have a sharp and rough personality, dull and smooth foods will help restore balance. It is really that simple. The key is to know which foods have the qualities that you need. The qualities that are found in a food are determined primarily by its taste. These qualities can then be altered through preparation and processing. This is the art of ayurvedic cooking.

The Six Tastes

Taste is what provides the nourishment of life. When a food tastes good, it is generally nourishing on at least some level. When it tastes bad, it is not likely that the food can sustain you. The body craves life-sustaining foods and we are drawn to them through our sense of taste. Interestingly, cravings can change dramatically from time to time. Foods that were once desirable may become undesirable. A person may really enjoy pizza and pasta but when they have the flu, they lose their taste for these foods.

Unfortunately, in the modern world, it is not easy to trust one's sense of taste. Through the processing and preparation of food, some foods that the body would not ordinarily crave become desirable. Modern technology has learned how to fool the senses, making unhealthy food taste good. With such an abundance of these foods around, the taste sense has begun to identify these foods as the norm and loses its ability to discern what is truly nourishing and harmonious from what is unhealthy and disharmonious. Lacking in discernment and desirous of pleasure, most people have become addicted to foods that eventually cause disease. Returning to a state of sensory discernment requires some re-education and inspiration, as well as the more difficult behavioral task of breaking the bad habits. Understanding the six tastes from an ayurvedic perspective begins the process of re-education.

Ayurveda divides up food into six tastes, each having its own set of qualities. Each taste is composed of two basic elements. The six tastes, their elemental makeup and their qualities affect the three doshas and your health.

As we explore the six tastes and, later, as we explore other treatments, you will see the symbols + or – following the letters V,P and K. V,P and K stand for each dosha. V is Vata. P is Pitta and K is Kapha. A + sign following a letter means that the dosha is increased. A – sign means that the dosha is decreased or balanced by the substance. So, when you see VP-K+ below for the sweet taste, it means that the sweet taste decreases or balances the vata and pitta doshas while increasing the kapha dosha. Thus, it is good for vata and pitta doshas but bad for kapha dosha. Sometimes you will see a (n) sign following a letter. This means that it has a virtually neutral effect on that dosha. Other times, you will see a + (ex) following a letter. This means that it will only increase and aggravate the dosha if it is consumed in excess. If you have a vata nature or imbalance, avoid V+. If you have a pitta nature of imbalance, avoid P+, if you have a kapha nature or imbalance, avoid K+.

The Sweet Taste (VP-K+)

The sweet taste is made up of earth and water. These are the same elements that make up the kapha dosha. Thus, when the sweet taste is taken into the body, all of the qualities of the kapha dosha increase. These qualities are: heavy, cool, moist, stable, dull, soft, gross, dense, smooth and cloudy. If these qualities are already in excess within you, then the sweet taste should be limited. For example; if you are overweight (heavy), mucusy (moist), dull or cloudy minded, or lethargic (stable), your diet should minimize the sweet taste. On the other hand, if you are underweight (light), anxious (mobile), critical (sharp), and so on, then the sweet taste is balancing for you.

In Ayurveda, when we talk about the sweet taste we are not talking about sugar and sugary treats. While sweet, most of these are overly processed and devoid of their natural nutrient value. These sweets are called simple carbohydrates in Western science. The ayurvedic concept of the sweet taste applies more closely to what Western science calls complex carbohydrates and fats. Positive examples of the sweet taste include most grains, milk, cheese, unsalted nuts and oils. By taking in more of these foods, the sweet taste and its qualities increase in the body and mind.

The sweet taste is the most nourishing of the six tastes. It supports strength and builds the tissues of the body. When the sweet taste is properly digested, it prevents disturbances within the vata and pitta doshas. When those doshas are out of balance, the sweet taste is a part of a complete program to restore health.

While being the most nourishing of the six tastes, it is heavy and difficult to digest. This is another reason why it should be taken in proper amounts. If it is not digested properly, the sweet taste has the greatest potential to create ama (toxins) in the body. To assure proper digestion, it is best to eat it properly according to the guidelines already mentioned and also to add some pungent spices to dishes that contain the sweet taste. These spices enhance digestion.

The Sour Taste (V-PK+)

The sour taste is made up of mostly fire and earth, with a little bit of water. Having the combined qualities of these elements, the sour taste is warm, heavy, moist, stable, sharp, soft, gross, flowing and cloudy. Taking in sour foods will increase these qualities in the body and mind. If digestion is a little weak, this taste can be helpful, because it supports the natural digestive fire, which is also warm and sharp. Being heavy, the sour taste also builds strength and body tissue. However, if a person has a hot and sharp personality (heated temper and critical tongue), taking in lots of these foods would only increase this aspect of their nature and create greater imbalance.

The sour taste is best for bringing balance to people with a vata nature or vata imbalance. It helps to bring stability to their digestive system and also helps to improve circulation. However, it is not recommended for people with a pitta nature or imbalance, as it is too hot and sharp, and it is also not very balancing for kapha, because it is too heavy, gross and cloudy. Examples of foods that have a sour taste are those which are fermented or cultured. These include yogurt, pickles, sauerkraut, tempe and sour plums. When foods are very sour, such as sauerkraut, they need only be taken in small amounts to improve digestion.

The Salty Taste (V-PK+)

The salty taste is made up of fire and water. These are the same elements that the pitta dosha is composed of. Thus, taking in the salty taste increases pitta and the qualities that it contains. The salty taste is hot, not heavy or light, slightly moist, mobile, sharp, clear, smooth, flowing, subtle and hard. Consuming more salt increases these qualities and increases pitta dosha. If appetite or digestion is weak, more salt can help, as it is warm and sharp, just like the fire that creates appetite and digestion. If the skin is rough, more salt can help it become smoother. If muscles are too hard and rigid, salt can help soften them and support flexibility.

In the West, salt has developed a bad reputation and many people have been advised to avoid it or reduce their intake. One reason is because salt can increase water retention and, as a result, increase blood pressure. However, this is not always the best advice. The salty taste helps bring balance to the vata dosha. Those of you with a vata nature or imbalance benefit from more salt and salty foods in your diet! This is because salt also helps to reduce fear and anxiety, moistens the skin, softens stools and it has a host of other beneficial properties that you will enjoy. This is not to say that you should take it in excessive amounts but you should also not overly reduce it. If you receive too little salt, your body and mind will become more rigid and fear and anxiety can actually increase!

A significant amount of salt is not beneficial for everyone. Salt increases the fiery qualities of the pitta dosha and the watery qualities of the kapha dosha. It makes pitta too hot and sharp and it makes kapha too soft and fluidic. If you have a pitta or kapha nature, reduce the amount of salt in your diet. Salty foods include seafood, seaweeds and of course, any dish that you add salt to.

The Bitter Taste (PK-V+)

The bitter taste is made of the air and ether elements. These are the same elements that the vata dosha is made up of and, as such, they share the same qualities. The bitter taste is cold, light, dry, mobile, sharp, hard, flowing, subtle, rough and clear. Eating foods with a bitter taste increases these qualities in the body and mind and increases the vata dosha. Taking in bitter-tasting foods is beneficial if a person has an excess of heat in their body. Being cold, the bitter taste antidotes the heat. The bitter taste also dries out the body, which is great if a person has an excessive secretion of oil on their skin or has acne. But it is not so good if a person has dry, rough skin or dry eyes. Because of its light quality, the bitter taste also supports weight loss, which is fine if there is obesity, but not so good if a person is underweight.

While the sweet taste is the most nourishing taste, the bitter taste is the most purifying. It helps to remove excess fat, ama and other toxins from the body. It purifies and removes excess heat from the liver and blood and also helps keep blood sugar levels within a normal range. Because many consider it unpleasant, it is not used as much as it could be in the diet and this has contributed to diabetes and obesity. Examples of foods with the bitter taste include a fruit called bitter melon and also many salad greens such as dandelion leaves, chard, kale and most green vegetable juices.

The bitter taste is most beneficial for those with a pitta nature, as it cools down the body and mind. It is also beneficial for kapha, as it is light and dry. Those with a vata nature or imbalance should take in only a minimal amount of the bitter taste, as it is too cold, dry and light.

The Pungent Taste: Hot-Spicy (K-PV+)

The pungent taste is made up of the elements air and fire. Air is a part of the vata dosha and fire is a part of the pitta dosha. So, it should come as no surprise that eating pungent foods increases these doshas. As the elements mix together, their combined qualities are hot, dry, light, mobile, sharp, hard, subtle, flowing, rough and clear. Taking in hot spicy (pungent) foods increases these qualities in the body and mind. Being hot, the pungent taste improves digestion and circulation, warms the body and sharpens the mind. However, if it is taken in excess, the hot quality can lead to anger and inflammation. And, while the dry quality is beneficial if there are excess secretions of mucus or oil, too much can create or exacerbate dry skin, turning it rough, and it can make the lungs overly dry and irritated.

Being the hottest of the six tastes, the pungent taste is very well known for increasing the strength and power of digestion. This makes it very beneficial for those with a kapha nature or imbalance. It improves the heavy feeling in the abdomen after eating and it supports weight loss. Although it works differently than the bitter taste, it purifies the body of excess fat and ama. The pungent taste is primarily taken in through hot spices such as ginger, black pepper, garlic, jalepeno, cayenne and other hot peppers. However, all spices have some pungency to them. Many leafy greens also have some pungency to them. The pungent taste is best for kapha but moderately spiced food is good for vata and mildly spiced food is beneficial for pitta.

The Astringent Taste (PK-V+)

The astringent taste is made up of the elements air and earth. The combined qualities of these two elements are cold, dry, stable, sharp, hard, dense, rough and cloudy. It is neither very heavy nor very light and it is neither gross nor subtle.

One of the most important and dramatic qualities of the astringent taste is its capacity to constrict and tone the tissues of the body. The earth element builds strength while, together, their dry quality makes tissues tight. The astringent taste makes the body firm, the joints stable and prevents the organs from sagging (prolapsing) as a person ages. Drooping organs occurs to some extent in everyone as they age, but it is often most noticeable in women, as the uterus can descend into the vaginal canal (uterine prolapse).

Because of its ability to increase body tone, the astringent taste is beneficial if there is joint hypermobility. However, if the body is stiff and inflexible, use of the astringent taste should be minimized. It is difficult to digest foods that are astringent. The dry and cold nature of the astringent taste weakens the digestive fire and dries up the secretion of digestive enzymes. Astringent-tasting foods often increase gas. In the mind, the contractive nature of the astringent taste has a limiting effect on the expansion of the mind and growth of awareness.

The best examples of the astringent taste are legumes such as lentils and beans. Most of these are very astringent and difficult to digest, resulting in excessive gas production. Because of its drying nature, the astringent taste should be avoided if you have a vata nature or imbalance. Because it is heavy, those with a kapha nature or imbalance should also avoid it. Only those with a pitta nature really benefit from astringent-tasting foods. Whenever astringent foods such as beans are taken, it is best to take them with a little oil and spice to improve digestibility.

The Best and Worst Tastes for Each Dosha

Each person requires all six tastes in order to be healthy. Each taste has its benefits to the body when it is taken in the proper amount. When taken in excess, each taste causes health challenges. The best meals have all of the tastes represented within them. However, the proper amount of each taste is determined by the constitution and the nature of the imbalances that are present. By taking in the six tastes, the body is assured of receiving the widest variety of nutrients. The art of ayurvedic nutrition is the art of properly balancing the six tastes.

Below are the tastes that are the best and the worst for each dosha. The best tastes balance the dosha and the worst tastes increase or aggravate the dosha, causing more problems. When you choose foods to eat, emphasize the tastes that balance the predominant dosha of your constitution and take only a small amount of the tastes that increase it. If you have an imbalance related to a specific dosha, avoid the foods that increase that dosha and increase the foods that bring it back to balance.

Dosha	Balance or Decrease (Best)	Increase (Worst)
Vata	Sweet, sour, salty	Bitter, pungent, astringent
Pitta	Sweet, bitter, astringent	Sour, salty, pungent
Kapha	Bitter, pungent, astringent	Sweet, sour, salty

The Benefits and Consequences of an Excess and Deficiency of Each Taste

Taste	Major Benefits	Excess	Deficiency
Sweet	Builds strength and tissues	Obesity, lethargy, diabetes, ama	Malnutrition, weak tissues
Sour	Promotes digestion	Hyperacidity, obesity, anger	Weak digestion, poor discrimination
Salty	Promotes appetite and flexibility	Water retention	Inflexibility of the body and mind
Pungent	Promotes digestion, purifies the body	Hyperacidity, weight loss, dry tissues, anger	Weak digestion, weight gain, lethargy, buildup of ama and mucus
Bitter	Purifies the body	Weight loss, anxiety, feeling cold, dry tissues	Weight gain, buildup of ama, acne
Astringent	Keeps the tissue tone	Inflexibility of the body and mind. Poor digestion	Loss of tissue tone, hypermobility

Basic Food Programs for the Three Doshas

The Vata Food Program

If you have a vata nature or imbalance and wish to heal yourself through diet, there are six important keys which, if followed, will make a profound difference in your health and well-being.

- Take food in small amounts
- Take food often
- Take foods at the same time each day
- Take foods that are heavier and nourishing
- Take foods that are moderately spiced
- Take food and drink that are warm

Take food in small amounts: The strength of the digestive system of a person with a vata nature or imbalance is usually weak. Think of a small fire in the belly. In order not to overwhelm the weak fire, only a small quantity of food should be taken at a time. If more is taken, gas, bloating or cramping can occur. How much is a small amount? That is not easy to say but suffice is to say that after eating, you should not feel heavy or full. As noted above under the proper guidelines for healthy eating, it is best to eat till only three-quarters full. It takes less to create this state in a person with a vata nature or imbalance. If you pay attention to how you feel as you are eating, you will know when you have reached that level.

Take food often: Since you can only digest well a small amount of food at a time, you can eat more often. This has many benefits, including keeping your blood sugar levels from falling too low, a common cause of irritability, anxiety and dizziness. By eating the proper foods in small amounts often, you will be assured of digesting the food well and building up your strength.

Take foods at the same time each day: Keeping a regular routine is very important. It is the nature of those with a vata imbalance to skip meals, eat at irregular times and, put simply, to have no routines what-so-ever. By taking foods at the same time each day, the mobile quality of vata dosha is reduced and stability returns. As a result, anxiety, worry and irritability are reduced and the strength of the digestion remains steady.

Take foods that are heavier and nourishing: Heavy and nourishing foods are those with a sweet and / or sour taste. Foods such as milk, yogurt, nuts and grains are best. Lighter foods, such as fruits and salads, should only be taken in small amounts. Interestingly, these heavy foods are the most difficult to digest. Thus, it is important that they are prepared with spices to assist digestion and taken in small amounts.

Take foods that are moderately spiced: One part of the proper preparation of food is to take it with the proper amount of spice. Those of you with a vata nature should add spices to your food to improve digestion. This is especially true when taking heavier foods. The overall effect of the spicing should be moderate and not too hot. Spices such as ginger, black pepper, cinnamon, cloves may be used. All spices are good for vata as long as they are not taken in excess. Nourishing foods should always be taken with some spice. Even milk can be prepared by warming it up with some ginger, cinnamon and cardamom in it. Spices improve both taste and digestion. If heavier foods are taken without spices, gas and bloating is pretty much assured, and ama will form.

Take food and drink that are warm: Warm foods support the digestive fire making them easier to digest. Cooked foods are better than raw foods for a person of vata imbalance for just this reason. Raw foods are generally cooler and suppress the fire. As a result, raw foods are more likely to produce gas and cramping. Even milk is best taken warm. Next time you go to a restaurant, ask for water with no ice. And, better yet, ask for some hot water to sip on while waiting for your meal. If you want to "spice" it up, ask for a slice of ginger and a squeeze of lemon to put in it.

The Pitta Food Program

If you have a pitta nature or imbalance and wish to heal yourself through diet, there are seven important keys, which, if followed, will make a profound difference in your health and well-being.

- Take food in moderate amounts

- Take three meals per day
- Take foods at the same time each day
- Balance nourishing foods with cleansing foods
- Take foods that are mildly spiced
- Avoid deep-fried foods
- Take food and drink at room temperature or warm, never hot

Take food in moderate amounts: A strong fire looks for something to burn. While having a strong digestive fire may mean that you digest food well, it also means that you will have a large appetite. Self-control is important. Make sure that you do not overeat. Eat only till you are 75% full. It is important to note that it takes a person of pitta nature a little longer to get to 75% than it does for people with other constitutions. This is because of the efficiency of their digestive system. People with a pitta nature can eat more than a person with a vata or kapha nature. How will you know when you've arrived? Pay attention. When hunger disappears and you are satisfied, you have arrived. You may want more, but you don't need more. Excess eating eventually suppresses digestion and metabolism, even though the appetite remains strong. This results in weight gain and the formation of ama (toxins due to poorly digested food). Indigestion can include burning, diarrhea and very smelly gas.

Take three meals per day: If your digestion is strong, take three satisfying meals per day, including breakfast, lunch and dinner. The key is to avoid snacking between meals and in the evening. Each meal should be large enough to hold you to the next meal. Lunch is the best time to take the largest meal, as digestion is the strongest at that time and you have the day ahead of you to digest it. Dinner should be quite a bit lighter, as there is not much time to digest it before you go to bed.

Take foods at the same time each day: This is less of a challenge for a person of pitta nature than a person of vata nature. As soon as there is little food left to digest in your stomach, the fire notifies you that it is time to eat and appetite rapidly increases. Eating at the same time each day trains the fire to know when food is coming and digestion quickly adapts to the schedule.

Balance nourishing foods with cleansing foods: When in balance and healthy, heavier and nourishing foods are most beneficial, as they build strength when properly digested. However, when excess heat builds up in the body (intensity, fever, feeling too warm) and when digestion has been compromised (when gas gets smelly), it is time to spend more time with cleansing foods. Nourishing foods are those that are heavier, such as milk and grains. Cleansing foods are those that are lighter, such as salads, soups, fruits and seeds.

Take foods that are mildly spiced: Mildly spiced foods improve digestion but do not overheat the body. This is particularly important when eating heavier foods, as they tend to naturally suppress the digestive fire. If not enough spice is taken, ama (toxins) form and kapha can increase, resulting in weight gain. Be careful though, too much spice easily aggravates pitta, producing more heat. Some spices, such as fennel, coriander, cardamom and peppermint, can be used in abundance. Others that are hotter, such as ginger, hot peppers, and hot mustards, should be taken only in the smallest amounts. In the end though, which spice is used is not as important as the end result you get when the food has been prepared and the spicing is complete. If the food tastes spicy hot, then it is too hot. The end result should be mild.

Avoid deep-fried foods: Deep-fried foods, especially at fast-food restaurants, are hot, salty and oily. This is the absolute worst combination for a person with a pitta imbalance. You may recall that pitta is made up of fire and water and is hot and moist. Deep-fried foods, such as French fries, onion rings and the like are filled with oil, suppress agni (digestive fire), and are hard to digest. Salt that is added to these foods only increases the aggravation to the pitta dosha. Deep-fried foods promote ama and increase kapha (weight).

Take food and drink at room temperature or warm, never hot: Having enough heat inside to begin with, more heat is not what you need. Cooked foods are warmer than raw foods and as such, raw foods are best for you, especially during the hot summer. This is a great time for large salads. Only during the winter are cooked foods advised, as their warmth is needed to antidote the cold weather. Drinks should be taken at room temperature or warm, but not hot. While it may seem logical that ice water would be beneficial, it is not. When drinks are taken too cold, your blood vessels constrict, and this prevents the heat that has built up inside from being released. As a result, the heat is pushed deeper within. Intense cold prevents heat from dispersing naturally. This is also a problem when walking from the heat of the outdoors into an air-conditioned room. If the change is too sudden, it becomes a source of stress and disturbs the normal functions of the body. When cooling down, it is best to do so gradually.

The Kapha Food Program
If you have a kapha nature or imbalance and wish to heal yourself through diet, there are seven important keys, which, if followed, will make a profound difference in your health and well-being.

- Take food in small amounts
- Take only two meals per day
- Take foods at the same time each day
- Take foods which are lighter and cleansing
- Take foods that are spiced hot
- Take foods and drinks that are hot
- Hold the oil: Avoid deep-fried foods and cream sauces

Take food in small amounts: For a person with a kapha nature, this is not so hard, as appetite is generally low. However, when a kapha imbalance combines with a pitta nature, appetite remains high even though weight has increased. When a kapha imbalance occurs in a person with a vata nature, the appetite may remain variable. Either way taking food in small amounts is important, because digestion is weak and the fire is low.

Take only two meals per day: Food is digested slowest in a person of kapha nature. True appetite takes a longer time to return. If you eat according to the traditional rhythm of three meals per day, you are very likely to gain weight. On a two meal per day schedule, it is best to take one of those for brunch at around 10:00 am and the last meal in the early evening around 5:00 or 6:00 pm.

Take foods at the same time each day: By taking the two meals at the same time each day, your body and your agni (digestive fire) will adjust to the rhythm of your appetite and the strength of your digestion will begin to increase at that time.

Take foods that are lighter and cleansing: Lighter, cleansing foods are those that help to rid the body of excess fat and ama (toxin). These foods include lots of vegetables, broths and seeds. Fruits, while light and cleansing, contain too much water and are not recommended in large amounts. If you take more of these foods and less of the heavier grains, dairy and nuts, your weight will return to normal and less mucous will be formed.

Take foods that are spiced hot: Spicing improves appetite and strengthens digestion. They also dry out the body. This is all very good for kapha. Having a consistently low digestive fire to begin with and excess water in the tissues, hot spices are a perfect addition to any meal. Hot peppers, mustards, ginger and black pepper are good examples of spices that should be added liberally to foods. Hot spices such as ginger, cinnamon and clove can also be taken as a beverage tea throughout the day.

Take foods and drinks that are hot: As those with a kapha constitution have a weak digestive fire, raw foods and cold drinks can make a bad situation worse. Drinks are best taken hot as a tea rather than at room temperature or cold out of the refrigerator. Emphasize cooked, well spiced foods in your diet that are served warm. In the summertime, however, when the temperature outside becomes very hot, raw salad greens are fine as they are light. However, because they are cooling, they are best taken with a light peppery dressing.

Hold the oil; avoid deep-fried foods and cream sauces: Oil and cream sauces (made up of water and earth) are simply not harmonious foods for you. These foods are heavy and moist and they suppress the fire, leading to weight gain, mucous formation and lethargy. By avoiding these foods, weight is reduced and less mucus is produced.

General Food Groups and their Effects on the Three Doshas

Long foods lists can be difficult to memorize and cumbersome to carry with you to every meal. By learning the basic effects of each food group, it becomes easier to make healthy choices. While within every food group there are exceptions, eating by food group will, for the most part, return you to a state of balance. When the chart states that a food group is balancing, make this food group a large part of your diet. Where the chart says increasing, make this group a small part of your food program. In general, it is best not to completely avoid any food group. For more specific details within each group, see the next food table.

	Basic Qualities	Vata	Pitta	Kapha
Grains	Heavy	Balancing	Balancing	Increasing
Milk and Cheese	Heavy, moist, cool	Balancing	Balancing	Increasing
Yogurt and other fermented milk products	Heavy, moist, warm	Balancing	Increasing	Increasing
Nuts	Heavy, moist, warm	Balancing	Slightly increasing	Increasing
Seeds	Light, dry	Increasing	Balancing	Balancing
Beans/Legumes	Heavy, dry	Increasing	Balancing	Increasing
Sweet Fruits	Light, moist, cool	Increasing	Balancing	Increasing
Sour Fruits	Light, moist, warm	Balancing	Increasing	Increasing
Root Vegetables	Heavy	Balancing	Balancing	Increasing
Leafy Vegetables	Light, dry	Increasing	Balancing	Balancing
*White Meat of fowl	Heavy, dry, cool	Increasing	Balancing	Increasing
* Dark Meat of fowl	Heavy, moist, warm	Balancing	Increasing	Increasing
*Eggs	Neutral	Balancing	Balancing	Balancing
Oils	Heavy, moist	Balancing	Slightly increasing	Increasing
White Sugar	Heavy, moist, mobile	Increasing	Increasing	Increasing
Fresh Honey/Molasses /Raw Sugar Cane	Heavy, moist, warm	Balancing	Increasing	**Increasing
Maple sugar/Maltose	Heavy, moist, cool	Increasing	Balancing	Increasing
Spices	Light, dry, warm	Balancing (moderate)	Balancing (mild)	Balancing (hot)

*Meat is not generally recommended as food source. Meat causes dullness within the body and mind and when taken for any reason other than for healing it is believed to interfere with spiritual awareness.

**Those with a kapha nature or imbalance can take modest amounts of older honey. Honey should be more than six months old. Older honey is drier and spicier.

Food Groups for the Three Doshas

This chart shows you which food groups are best for each dosha and those that are likely to lead to imbalance, especially if they are overeaten. Take a larger amount of food from the best list and take less from those on the worst list. In general, do not completely avoid any food as variety is important.

	Best	Worst
Vata	Grains, milk, cheese, nuts, sour fruits, root vegetables, dark meat of fowl, eggs, oils, fresh honey, raw sugar, spices	Leafy vegetables, white meat of fowl, white sugar, maple sugar/maltose
Pitta	Grains, milk, cheese, seeds, legumes, sweet fruits, root vegetables, leafy vegetables, white meat of fowl, egg, maple sugar/maltose	Yogurt and fermented dairy, nuts, sour fruits, dark meat of fowl, oils, white sugar, honey, molasses and raw sugars, hot spices
Kapha	Seeds, leafy vegetables, old honey, hot spices	Grains, milk, cheese, fermented dairy, nuts, sweet and sour fruits, root vegetables, white and dark meats of fowl, oils, sugars

Specific Foods within Each Food Group for Each Constitution

The following are specific food lists for each dosha. Those foods listed as balancing can be taken freely as a substantial part of a food program. Those listed as aggravating should be avoided except on rare occasions, as they can cause an imbalance. Those listed as mildly increasing may cause a slight imbalance but because their action is not very strong, they can be taken in small amounts daily or larger amounts once in a while. They should not be used in large amounts on a regular basis and if you are ill, they are best avoided.

The Vata Food List

Food Group	Vata Balancing	Mildly Vata Increasing	Strongly Vata Aggravating
Grains	Amaranth, oats (cooked), quinoa, rice (white or brown), wheat	Barley, millet	Buckwheat, corn flour (chips, bread and tortillas), dry oats (granola), polenta, rye
Dairy	Butter, buttermilk, kefir, milk, sour cream, yogurt (fresh)	Hard cheeses	Ice cream, frozen yogurt
Milk Alternatives	Almond milk, rice milk, oat milk	Soy milk	
Sweeteners	Raw, uncooked honey, jaggery (raw sugar), maltose, molasses, rice syrup, sucanat	Date sugar, grape sugar, maple syrup	Brown sugar, white sugar
Oils	Almond, ghee (clarified butter), sesame	Avocado, castor, coconut, flaxseed, mustard, peanut, sunflower	Safflower
Fruits	Baked apples, apricots, avocados, bananas (ripe), blackberries, cantaloupe, cherries, coconut, cranberry sauce, dates (not dry), figs (fresh), grapefruit, grapes, lemons, mangos, nectarines, oranges, papaya, peaches, pears, persimmons, pineapple, plums, raspberries, strawberries (ripe), tangerines	Apples, pomegranate	Dried fruit of any kind, cranberries
Vegetables	Avocado, beets, carrots (not as a juice), leeks, mustard greens, okra, onions (well cooked), parsnips, shallots, acorn squash, winter squash, sweet potatoes, tomatoes, water chestnuts	Broccoli, cauliflower, celery, corn, cucumber, eggplant, green beans, kale, medium chilies and hot peppers, mushrooms, potatoes, radishes, seaweed, spinach, sweet peas, zucchini. The following may be eaten uncooked with a creamy or oily dressing: lettuce, spinach, and any leafy green (occasional use only and with a spicy heavy dressing)	
Nuts	Almonds	Cashews, filberts, pecans, piñon, pistachio, and any other nut not mentioned	Peanuts
Seeds	Poppy	Pumpkin, sesame, sunflower	
Meat/Poultry/Eggs	Chicken and turkey (dark meat), beef, duck, eggs, lamb, pork, venison	Chicken and turkey (white meat)	
Fish	Fresh water fish, seafood	Shellfish	
Legumes	Split mung beans	Tofu, hummus, whole mung beans	Aduki beans, black beans, whole chickpeas, fava beans, kidney beans, lentils, Mexican beans, navy beans, pinto beans, soybeans (except as tofu)
Spices	All spices except those listed as mild	Black pepper, cayenne pepper, hot mustard	
Condiments	Mayonnaise, vinegar	Catsup	Carob, chocolate
Beverages	Water, spicy herbal teas	Diluted fruit juices	Alcohol, coffee, black or green tea, coffee, mineral water, fruit juices, soft drinks

The Pitta Food List

Food Group	Pitta Balancing	Mildly Pitta Increasing	Strongly Pitta Aggravating
Grains	Barley, white basmati rice, millet, oats, white rice, wheat, whole wheat	Brown rice	Buckwheat, corn flour
Dairy	Unsalted butter, cottage cheese, cream cheese, ghee, milk	Hard, non-salted cheeses	Buttermilk, salted cheeses, sour cream, kefir, cultured milks, yogurt
Milk Alternatives	Oat milk, soy milk, rice milk	Almond milk	
Sweeteners	Maltose, maple syrup, rice syrup	Dextrose, fructose, fresh honey, table sugar	Molasses, raw sugar, old honey
Oils	Ghee, olive oil	Avacado, canola, corn, coconut, soy, sunflower	Almond, castor, flaxseed, margarine, mustard, safflower, sesame
Fruits	Apples, avacados, blackberries, blueberries, cantaloupe, coconut, cranberries, dates, dried fruit, figs, grapes, lemons, limes, nectarines, pineapple, prunes, raisins, raspberries, strawberries	Apricots, bananas (very ripe only), cherries, grapefruit, oranges, pineapple	All sour fruits, such as sour oranges (mandarin), sour pineapple, sour plums, papaya, olives, tangerines, bananas and all unripe fruit
Vegetables	Alfalfa sprouts, artichoke, asparagus, bean sprouts, bell peppers, bitter melon, broccoli, Brussels sprouts, cabbage, cauliflower, celery, cilantro, cress, cucumber, green peppers, kale, leafy greens, lettuce, mushrooms, onions (well cooked), peas, pumpkin, seaweed, squash, zucchini	Avocado, beets, carrots, corn, eggplant, garlic (well cooked), parsley, potatoes, spinach, sweet potatoes, vine-ripened tomatoes	Chilies, hot peppers, mustard greens, onion (raw), radishes, tomato paste, tomato sauce and any hot or pungent vegetable
Nuts	Coconut	Pine nuts	Almonds, Brazil nuts, cashews, filbert, macadamia nuts, pecans, pistachio, peanuts, and any other nut not mentioned
Seeds	Sunflower, pumpkin	Sesame	
Meat/Poultry/Eggs	Chicken, egg whites, turkey	Beef, duck, egg yolk, lamb, pork, venison, any other red meat	
Fish	Fresh water fish (trout)	Sea fish	
Legumes	Black lentils, chickpeas, mung beans, split peas, soybeans (soy products), tofu	Aduki beans, kidney beans, navy beans, pinto beans	Red and yellow lentils
Spices	Cardamom, catnip, chamomile, coconut, coriander, dill, fennel, lemon verbena, peppermint, saffron, spearmint, turmeric	Basil, bay leaf, black pepper, caraway, cinnamon, cumin, ginger (fresh), oregano, rosemary, thyme	Anise, asafoetida, cayenne pepper, cloves, fenugreek, garlic (raw), ginger (dry), horseradish, hyssop, marjoram, mustard seeds, nutmeg, poppy seeds, sage, star anise
Condiments	Carob (only if sweetened with the best sweeteners above)	Mayonnaise, sweet mustards	Chocolate, salt, vinegar
Beverages	Water, bitter or astringent herb teas (alfalfa, chicory, dandelion, hibiscus, strawberry leaf), milk, wheat grass juice	Green or black tea (green is better), diluted fruit juice with one-half water	Alcohol, carbonated water, coffee, sweet fruit juices, spicy herb teas, soft drinks, tomato juice

The Kapha Food List

Food Group	Kapha Balancing	Mildly Kapha Increasing	Strongly Kapha Aggravating
Grains	Amaranth, barley, buckwheat, corn flour, quinoa	Millet, rye, basmati rice	Oats, long and short grain rice (white or brown), wheat, whole wheat
Dairy	Goat milk, skim milk	2% milk	Butter, buttermilk, cheese, cream, cottage cheese, ice cream, kefir, sour cream, yogurt, whole milk
Milk Alternatives		Almond milk, rice milk, soy milk	Oat milk
Sweeteners	Raw honey that is more than six months old	Raw honey that is less than six months old	Fructose, maple syrup, molasses, raw sugar, white and brown sugar
Oils	Canola, corn, flaxseed, mustard, safflower, soy, sunflower		Almond, avocado, castor, coconut, olive, peanut, sesame
Fruits	Dried fruits if not too sweet. Apple, cherries, cranberries, grapefruit, pomegranate, prunes, raisins	Apricots, lemon, lime, papaya, pineapple	Sweet fruits, avocado, bananas, berries (raspberry, blackberry, blueberry, strawberry), cantaloupe, coconut, dates, figs, grapes, mango, melons, pineapple, oranges, peaches, pears, persimmons, plums, tangerines, watermelon
Vegetables	Alfalfa sprouts, artichoke, asparagus, green beans, bell peppers, broccoli, Brussels sprouts, cabbage, cauliflower, carrots, celery, chilies, cilantro, corn, kale, lettuce, and other leafy greens, mustard greens, onions, parsley, peas, hot peppers, potatoes, radish, seaweed, spinach, rutabagas/turnips	Mushrooms, tomatoes	Beets, cucumber, eggplant, okra, squash (all), sweet potatoes, water chestnuts, zucchini
Nuts			Almonds, Brazil nuts, cashews, coconut, filberts, macadamia nuts, pecans, pistachio, peanuts, walnuts
Seeds	Pumpkin seeds, sunflower seeds	Sesame seeds	Lotus seeds, poppy seeds
Meat/Poultry/Eggs	Chicken or turkey (dark meat only), rabbit	Egg	All other meat and poultry
Fish	River fish		Seafood, shellfish
Legumes	Mung beans, red lentils, soybeans (tofu and soymilk), split peas	Aduki beans, black gram, black beans, fava beans, kidney beans, lima beans, pinto beans	Black lentils, chickpeas
Spices	Anise, basil, bay leaf, black pepper, calamus, chamomile, caraway, cardamom, catnip, cayenne, cinnamon, cloves, coriander, cumin, dill, fennel, fenugreek, garlic, ginger, horseradish, hyssop, marjoram, mustard, nutmeg, oregano, peppermint, poppy seeds, rosemary, saffron, sage, spearmint, star anise, thyme, turmeric. Hot spices are best.		Salt
Condiments		Catsup, vinegar	Mayonnaise, salt
Beverages	Water, herb teas (spicy and bitter), cranberry juice, green vegetable juices, wheat grass juice, green tea	Carbonated mineral water, coffee, black tea	Alpple juice, carrot juice, orange juice, soft drinks

Food Combining

In the grand scheme of healing your digestive system and your diet, proper food combining, although important, comes in last relative to how you eat your food and your overall food choices. In fact, if your digestion is strong and healthy, only the most insulting combinations will cause digestive upset. However, if after correcting how you eat and what you eat, you are still having challenges, then adding the rules of proper food combining into your food program can be very beneficial for correcting your digestive problems. Below are a few important rules taken from both ayurvedic and Western concepts of food combining.

Summary of the Rules of Proper Food Combining

- Bitter salads should be eaten at the end of a meal
- Astringent teas such as black tea or raspberry tea do not combine well with any food
- Strong sweets do not combine well with any other food; take them between meals if at all.
- When digestion is difficult, mixing two concentrated carbohydrates or two high protein foods should be avoided

Bitter Salads Taken at the End of a Meal: Salads are served cold and many of the ingredients are bitter and astringent. These tastes dry up digestive secretions and reduce the strength of the digestive fire. For this reason, if heavy food is taken after a salad, the heavier, harder-to-digest food is more likely to be poorly digested. Salads do not harm the digestion of food taken previously as that food being "ahead" in the line of digestion is unaffected.

Astringent Teas do not Combine Well with any Food: The astringent taste dries up secretions. This includes the secretion of digestive enzymes. Thus, if food is taken with or just after tea, it may be poorly digested. Astringent teas include black and green tea as well as some herbal teas such as raspberry. You will know if the tea is astringent if the roof of your mouth and perhaps your cheeks feel just a little tight after drinking it.

Strong Sweets do not Combine Well with Other Foods: Strong sugary sweet treats, sweet juices and sweet beverages of any kind disturb the digestion of the foods they are taken with. The sweet taste dominates the digestive process, shifting the process of digestion in favor of the sugar. This may be because sugar is so vital for life. However, any other food taken at the same time is often poorly digested. Thus, it is best to take sweet foods and drinks between meals, if you take them at all. What should you drink with your meals? A half cup of room temperature or warm water is best. If you like more flavor, add some lemon or lime.

Avoid Mixing Two Concentrated Carbohydrates or Two Concentrated Proteins Together: Sensitive digestive systems often find it difficult to digest steak and eggs together or fish and chicken. Likewise, potatoes and rice can be difficult. The most sensitive digestive systems benefit from taking just one of these types of foods at a time.

Last But Not Least

If you are taking food properly as outlined above and you are choosing the proper foods for your constitution and the current imbalance, you are very likely to be digesting your food well with little trouble. My own experience is that 95% of my patients see great reduction in gas, indigestion, bloating and diarrhea from this alone. In the patients who do not improve, I recommend also following the rules of proper food combining. This brings the results up to 99%. The last 1% is often due to deep-seated emotional challenges creating ongoing states of stress or significant digestive disease that has been present for several years, such as ulcerative colitis, Chron's disease or diverticulitis. However, even these patients dramatically improve after several weeks following this program.

There is one final rule and it applies to everyone with any type of significant digestive imbalance. There are some foods that are just very difficult to digest, except in the person with a very balanced digestive system. These foods are below. They should be avoided until digestion returns to normal.

Avoid the following difficult-to-digest foods:

- All beans, except well-cooked split mung beans
- Cruciferous vegetables (broccoli, cauliflower, kale, Brussels sprouts, cabbage)
- Deep-fried foods
- Concentrated sweet desserts (candy, cake, chocolates and any combination of flour, butter and sugar).

Some Final Thoughts on Digestion

It may seem like a lot to eat food properly, choose the proper foods and combine them together properly. Don't let the journey ahead overwhelm you. Even if you just improve a few habits, you can see remarkable improvement. Our clinic has treated many thousands of patients and, more than any other modality, I have seen the most dramatic results occur from the simplest dietary changes. Most people look outside of themselves for a cure. The cure for indigestion will never be found in a tablet. The most any pharmaceutical medicine can do is partially compensate for your disharmonious habits. That is a long way from healing your life. So start slowly and know that you have the rest of your life to continue mastering these principles.

Personal Reflections

Like you, I have struggled with my diet. I haven't always eaten healthy and there is still room for improvement as, like everyone to some extent, I struggle with desire. Over the years, I seem to be overcoming more and more of the struggles. When I was a child, I would sometimes eat a pint of ice cream at night for entertainment while watching television. If ice cream was not available, cookies usually were. I didn't eat just one, I finished the box. I grew up eating at MacDonald's, Burger King and Kentucky Fried Chicken. Fortunately, I was also an active athlete and so I burned off a lot of those calories and kept my weight down. But, when high school ended and I became more sedentary, my habits caused my weight to increase and I gained 20 pounds over the next 15 years. I became conscious of my weight and tried to use discipline but more often than not, I failed.

Having gone into the healing profession, I was more motivated to keep my weight down and look healthy. After all, it is hard to teach about health when you yourself are overweight. So I was quite determined, and still I struggled. When I turned 35, I gained 10 more pounds as my metabolism began to slow down. I am not very tall. Ok, I'm short, only 5'6". A gain of 30 pounds on someone who should be 145 pounds is worse than a gain of 30 pounds on someone who should be 200 pounds. I also knew where I was heading. My father was pushing 200 pounds and was the same size as me, with a similar constitution and metabolism. I have been determined not to let that happen to me. When I turned 42, something shifted in my consciousness and I decided that being 175 pounds was no longer acceptable.

I was already living what most people would consider a very healthy ayurvedic lifestyle. At that time I had been a vegetarian for nearly ten years and I ate foods that were for the most part pitta pacifying (Pitta being my predominant dosha). I said grace before my meals, ate sitting down and had given up cold drinks long ago. I followed most of the guidelines for healthy eating. Still, I was slowly gaining weight!

A little more self-study and honesty revealed to me that the reason I was overweight was two-fold. First, I ate too much sugar. I only wish that sugar came from killing animals; then I could morally object to eating it! Unfortunately, most sweet treats fit nicely into a vegetarian diet. In addition to the desserts, a large amount of sugar finds its way in most of our beverages except for water. The addition of sugar to foods or drinks has become so commonplace that our capacity to taste and enjoy food without large amounts of added sugar has been diminished. We are people addicted to sugar. But I digress. The second cause was that I simply ate too much. The size of my portions was too large. I took in much more than I needed and what I didn't need turned to fat. For the most part, portions in the United States are out of control. A wrap prepared at our local healthy café is large enough for two meals! It may be organic but it is still too much! The state of our beverages is no different.

A small coffee drink or sweetened tea at just about any café is 12 oz. That is really a cup and a half. A medium is 16 oz. That is two cups. A large is about 20-24 oz. That is nearly 3 cups. Take two of those each day and it adds up to a lot of extra calories and, over the course of a year, a lot of extra pounds. Don't get me started on the extra large soda drinks available at convenience stores. But I digress.

I had a very healthy lifestyle. But I ate and drank too much. I drank two to three 16 oz. cups of chai tea each day. I ate the portions served to me at restaurants and when I ate my wife's wonderful (and healthy) cooking, I went back for a second and sometimes a third portion.

When my consciousness finally shifted, I began valuing small portions. I'd even ask for a child-size portion! That size is closer to a normal healthy adult portion for someone my size with my metabolism. When I go out to eat now, I look for a meal my wife is willing to split with me. Sometimes we even just order nice appetizers. When I eat dinner at home, I now control my own portions.

It took two more years after I mastered portion control before I was ready for my next step – control over sugar intake. Of course, I had reduced my sugar intake by reducing my portions but there was still the afternoon cookie or muffin and the evening dessert. When it comes to sugary treats, I find moderation quite difficult. So, I broke the addiction cold turkey. Of course, it took me 45 years to get ready! After a year of no sugar passing my lips, I am now better able to moderate my sugar intake though it is a slippery slope.

By eating a healthy, reasonably portioned breakfast, lunch and dinner and reducing the size of my cups of chai tea lattes, I began to see the pounds shrink away. When I gave up refined sugars, I saw even more weight disappear. Today, I have lost 20 of the 30 pounds I put on since I was an athlete in high school and I have kept it off for four years.

For each of us, there are areas in which we can improve our relationship with food. Already choosing healthy foods and for the most part eating them properly, my next step was to reduce my intake, learn to eat only till I was 75% full and then to give up sugar. What is your next step? Remember that you have your whole life to master your health. Is your consciousness ready to change? That is the big question. Changes made one at a time, integrated into your lifestyle, are sustainable.

The key to making changes is conscious awareness. You have to be able to hear your own internal higher wisdom. Whether your challenge is gas and bloating, irritable bowel syndrome, or being overweight, you have to want it to be different. The logic that it makes sense to make changes is not enough. Your sensory desires work against your reasoning and win almost every time. To master your senses requires being able to listen to your soul's voice. Ayurveda and yoga teach that when the mind is quiet, we can hear the whispering of our

LESSON 10: HEALING YOUR LIFE THROUGH AROMATHERAPY

Walk in the woods after a fresh light rain,
the aromatic molecules of nature's children
dance in the air; playful, grounded and alive.

Like our sense of taste, through our sense of smell we take into our body, mind and consciousness impressions that can either lead to health and wellness or to disease. Most people don't think of their nose as a vehicle through which we take in anything important other than air but what is in that air is very important. Not all air is the same.

The air we breathe consists typically of 99 percent nitrogen and oxygen. The other one percent includes carbon dioxide, argon and other trace gases such as hydrogen, helium, neon and methane and even smaller amounts of carbon monoxide, ozone and nitrous oxide. Mixed in to all of this, dependent upon the humidity are water molecules. While these are the standard constituents of air, localized air often contains many other molecules. If you live near certain industrial plants, there will be releases of nitrogen, hydrogen sulfide and sulfuric acid into the air you breathe. If you live on the windward side of a mountain near a large population center, there will be excessive ozone in the air, a well-known irritant to the respiratory system. If you live in the city, automobiles increase the amount of carbon monoxide in your air. If you live near a coal power plant, you are likely breathing in excessive sulfur oxides and sulfur dioxide. In addition to the toxic constituents of air gifted to us by the industrial age are those that are gifted to us by our neighbors who smoke and who burn their garbage or brush. The air we breathe is full of chemicals. These chemicals enter our lungs. Some irritate the membranes of the lungs and cause localized damage. Others are absorbed into the bloodstream through the capillaries that pass nearby and are distributed to each of the tissues of our bodies. Many of these chemicals react within our bodies. Some of these reactions are known to result in inflammation and others in cancer.

While the localized air we breathe may be filled with unwanted molecules that cause harm, the air can be filled with many other molecules that you may appreciate. Our aromatic environment is also chemically based. These chemicals are often referred to as phytochemicals and our localized air may be filled with them. Examples are the aromatic constituents of lavender, rosemary, roses, grasses, moist soil, pine and so much more. These phytomolecules also enter your body through your capillary system and participate in biochemical reactions. Exactly how they participate in biochemical reactions within the body is still not well understood. But, they do act and simple observation can tell you that their actions are not just physical but emotional. Practitioners of aromatherapy understand that, in addition to absorption into the bloodstream, these phytochemicals stimulate various nerve receptors within the nasal cavity and sinuses sending signals directly to different parts of the brain, including the limbic system. Neuroscientists believe that this is the region of our brains that process emotion and memory.

While we may like to think that all phytochemicals that we inhale are good for us and all industrial chemicals are bad, it is not that simple. Ayurveda teaches us that nothing is healthy for everyone and nothing is harmful to everyone. What we take in through our sense of smell can best be described as either harmonious or disharmonious.

On the gross level, if we breathe in toxins, we will obviously become physically sick. Some of those toxins, such as nerve gas, are strong and powerful and quickly cause harm. Most toxins, however, are subtler but can still cause significant discomfort. Some people have a strong reaction to smelling chemical perfumes, fresh paint or road tar. Common reactions include headaches, stomachaches, dizziness and confusion.

Each day we breathe in thousands of chemicals and each has some effect upon us. Some people are more sensitive to these chemicals that others. Those who are highly sensitive are considered to suffer from a condition called Multiple Chemical Sensitivity Syndrome (MCSS). People with this diagnosis react dramatically to even very low levels of exposure. Common symptoms of MCCS include runny nose, itchy eyes, headaches, scratchy throat, earaches, mental confusion, sleepiness, stomachaches, nausea and aching joints. Some people even have strong symptoms that are completely debilitating.

Even if you don't have MCSS, you still react to the world around you through your sense of smell. Some of these reactions may be bothersome, but most of the time, we are not conscious of the effect that smells have on us. This does not mean, however, that their effect is insignificant. Smells most often affect our mood without us even knowing.

If you walk through a flower garden and smell the jasmine, lavender and roses, how does it make you feel? How does the smell of the earth when the rains begin make you feel? Does the smell of fresh baked bread or the preparation of food in the kitchen evoke any feelings? We are constantly surrounded by aromas. Food in the restaurants, popcorn in the movie theater, flowers in the garden, perfumes on other people, scented products that we put on our bodies, coffee, tea, roadwork, paint, carpets, and the list goes on and on. Living the world is an aromatic experience!

Our emotions are never separate from the environment. While some of what is experienced through our sense of smell is purely chemical, some is the result of associations we have made with past experiences, pleasant or unpleasant.

A particular scent can bring back memories long forgotten and the emotions associated with them. An adult who grew up in a loving baker's family may experience a greater sense of security and relaxation in the home of someone baking bread many years later.

Healing your life through your sense of smell means taking conscious control over your aromatic environment. It means choosing aromas that support your well-being. Depending upon your constitution and the nature of any imbalances within you, the proper aromas can be selected that support helping you to return to balance.

Aromas, being a part of nature, are made up of the five elements and can be understood in terms of the ten pairs of opposite qualities. Knowing your own qualities and the qualities of the aromas allows you to create a supportive environment.

Most aromas used in aromatherapy come from plant oils. These oils can be found in any part of a plant. Rose oil comes from a flower, frankincense from a resin and cinnamon from bark or leaf. Conscious aromatherapy can be created by either keeping supportive plants nearby or by purchasing the aromatic, essential oils of the plant and using them appropriately.

The Elemental Qualities of Oils

Just like foods, essential oils have qualities that are either suited for an individual or contribute to an imbalance. Every scent is made up of some combinations of the five elements. As a result, they have their own unique combinations of the ten pairs of opposite qualities. Knowing the major qualities of the aroma will tell you a lot about its effects on the mind. Clues to the elemental makeup of an aromatic scent and its qualities are found in an oil's taste and also in the part of the plant used to make the essential oil. Each of the six tastes (sweet, sour, salty, pungent, bitter, astringent) can be identified in certain aromas. While we don't physically taste the aroma, we use the same terminology of the six tastes to describe the aromatic experience.

All aromas have a generally subtle, light and flowing quality. This is because the element ether predominates in all aromas. The etheric qualities of aromas allow them to waft through the air, expanding their influence outward until their aromatic qualities dissipate. Since ether is predominant in all aromas, to some degree, all aromas increase the vata dosha. This is particularly true when aromatic qualities are very strong. While aromas exist within a field of ether, other elements and their qualities mix with ether to create the overall effect.

When ether combines with the fire element, an aroma becomes heating. This occurs with aromas that have a pungent, sour or salty quality. The essential oils of calamus, clove, basil, eucalyptus and ginger are examples of oils with a pungent aroma. Fish oils and seaweeds have a salty, sea-like aroma. The sour aroma is found in sour fruits and berries. As a result, they have warm, sharp and stimulating qualities in addition to being light and flowing. Because of their fire, these oils and their aromas aggravate the pitta dosha.

When ether mixes with the air element, the effect becomes more mobile and this creates stimulation and agitation. Physically, it causes the heart rate to increase; mentally, the mind moves more quickly; and emotionally, there can occur an increase in anxiety. Aromas that are bitter and pungent have more air in them and can create these effects. Examples of aromas that are both pungent and bitter and thus contain the most air are vetiver, calamus and patchouli. These aromas are best for bringing balance to the kapha dosha but can aggravate the vata dosha.

When the water element mixes with ether, the aroma becomes cooler, softer and smoother. It is more nourishing, increases compassion and softens emotions. It helps to heal the heart of emotional hurt while increasing a person's desire for life. Physically, it helps to moisten the skin. When the water element enters into an aroma, the aroma becomes sweeter. Examples include rose, lily, lotus and saffron.

When the earth element mixes with ether, an aroma becomes cooler and heavier. Aromas that are sweet or astringent have a greater amount of earth within them. These aromas help to ground, calm and stabilize the mind reducing anxiety and worry. Examples include the woody aromas such as sandalwood, agarwood and cedarwood. Essential oils that are collected from the root of a plant also have more earth element within the aroma. This includes ginger, valerian and vetiver. Their heavier quality is an antidote for being light-headed.

The Parts of a Plant / Sources of Essential Oils

Essential oils can be gathered from almost any part of the plant. However, not all parts of the plant have the same concentration of oil. In addition, the biochemistry of the different parts of a plant can vary, making their aromatic qualities different as well. The common parts of the plant that oils are collected from are as follows:

Roots: Direct contact with the earth brings about an earthier aromatic quality. As the earth element is a part of the astringent and sweet tastes, oils from these parts of the plant often have these aromatic tastes. As a result of their connection to the earth, they are heavier and more stable. This makes them better for those with a vata or pitta nature and not very good for those with a kapha nature. Of course, within a root, other elements may mix with these qualities, altering their final presentation. Examples of root plants from which oils are collected are ginger, turmeric, valerian and vetiver.

Heartwood and Trunk: The heartwood of a plant is the wood found below the bark toward the center of a tree. Like the stem of a plant, it circulates fluids and nutrients and is hard, heavy and stable. As a result, it has more earth and water elements within it and a sweet, woody aroma. Oils from this part of the plant are generally best for vata and pitta and are not as good for kapha dosha. Of course, within the stem, other elements may uniquely mix with these qualities, altering their final presentation. Examples of oils collected from the heartwood of trees include cedarwood and agarwood.

Bark: The bark of a tree is woody and hard. Unlike the heartwood, circulation does not strongly occur here and as a result it is drier and contains less water. The earth element is predominant. Oils from the bark of a tree are heavy, stabilizing and protective. They have a sweet or astringent aroma to them. Of course, within the bark, other elements may uniquely mix with these qualities, altering their final presentation. Examples of oils that can be collected from bark include birch, cinnamon and prickly ash.

Resin: A tree resin in a thick fluidic sap that is excreted by a tree usually in response to stress or injury often created by bug infestations or cutting the tree. Tree resin helps the tree to heal the wound and also protects it against infestations. Likewise, resins are often applied to the skin to aid in the healing of wounds. Many are also antiseptic. Often collected from the bark, most resins are described as combining the qualities of astringency with a sweet, woody quality. They have an overall drying effect on the skin and, as a result, are used in small areas. However, their strong aromatic quality permeates the surrounding area and is often quite pleasant. Examples of resins that are collected for their oil include frankincense and myrrh.

Leaves: The leaf of a plant is more fragile than the parts previously mentioned. Growing high upon the plant and opening themselves to the sky, they contain more air. This is particularly true of those that grow in the shade. Those that grow in full sun will take on some of its fiery characteristics. As a result, leaves tend to have a more bitter or pungent aromatic quality. Of course, within the leaf, other elements may uniquely mix with these qualities, altering their final presentation. Examples of oils commonly collected from leaves include bay, cinnamon, eucalyptus, mint and patchouli.

Flowers: The flower of the plant is the most delicate part of the plant. It grows furthest from the root and reaches toward the heavens. It contains the most ether of any part of the plant and, as a result, has a generally light quality that is uplifting and inspiring. Some flowers have little scent. Those that have a stronger floral scent owe it to a mix of other elements into the field of ether. The scent of the most desirable flowers is sweet owing to the addition of a watery element. Some have a secondary pungency as fire enters the mix. Because of its strong ether content, even when water is present, the floral scent remains light and delicate. Of course, within the flower, other elements may uniquely mix with the ether, altering its final presentation. Examples of oils collected from flowers include rose, jasmine, clary sage and lily.

Different Types of Aromatic Oils

A little background can be helpful to understand the myriad of aromatic choices that are available on the store shelves. There are four basic types: Essential Oils, Hydrosols, Absolutes and Attars.

An essential oil is a distinctive volatile oil of a plant that carries its aromatic essence. It is usually produced by steam distillation and is free of chemicals. Steam passes through the plant material in closed environment. The steam causes the volatile oils to evaporate and mix with the steam. The steam is then condensed into a liquid containing the essential oil. Some essential oils prepared in this manner include the name Otto on the label, such as Rose Otto.

A hydrosol is prepared from the recondensed steam after the distillation process is complete. The water retains some of the aromatic qualities of the plant. Rose hydrosol is very popular and may be used as a spray mister applied to the face and body.

An absolute is prepared from a chemical distillation process that most often uses carbon dioxide, hexane and alcohol. These are less expensive than those produced by steam distillation. As absolutes retain some chemical impurities they cost less and are considered to be inferior by aromatherapists.

An attar is an oil that is prepared by merging the properties of an essential oil into sandalwood oil. The resulting combination is often less expensive than the essential oil.

Blending Essential Oils—Have Fun!

It is not always possible to receive all of the qualities that you need to balance yourself from one essential oil. This is why blending oils can be very helpful. Blending oils is also fun. You should approach the making of oil blends as a time of play. Add a drop of the essential oil to the base oil and see how you like it. Then add more. Mix in another. See how the aromatic qualities change as you add another drop. The end result is not only based upon each ingredient but upon how much of each you add. Write down what you do because if you stumble upon a blend you really like, it is a shame if you can't recreate it. Dozens of essential oils can be found in almost any natural food store. Just like making soup, any oil can be added to a blend. The final blend should be assessed for its qualities. Below are a few ideas for each dosha.

Vata Dosha

Those with a vata nature are supported by oils and blends that are warming and calming. The combination of sweet and spicy oils is particularly beneficial. The sweeter oils are nourishing and the spicy oils are warming. Essential oils of sandalwood and chamomile are sweet and calming but they are also cooling. So adding a small amount of cinnamon to the mix makes for a perfect blend.

Pitta Dosha

Those with a pitta nature are supported by oils that are cooling. Many sweet floral fragrances, such as rose, jasmine and honeysuckle, are cooling. They also combine well together. Sandalwood and frankincense are additional cooling oils and are woodier and more grounding.

Kapha Dosha

Those with a kapha nature are supported by warm and stimulating oils and blends. Oils of patchouli, clove and cinnamon are all warm and stimulating and combine well together.

Selected Essential Oils for Each Dosha

Vata	Pitta	Kapha
Sandalwood	Sandalwood	Clove
Jasmine	Rose	Patchouli
Lavender	Lavender	Cinnamon
Chamomile	Honeysuckle	Sage
Cinnamon	Lily	Basil
Rosemary	Frankincense	Cedar

Essential Oils and the Mind

The intake of aromatic scents occurs through the intake of tiny molecules through your nose, which enter into your sinuses and are then perceived by nerve endings that lead to your brain. In addition, a small but powerful amount of these tiny molecules are absorbed directly into the blood supply and circulate to the brain. The end result is a quick, almost immediate adjustment to your mood. Conscious aromatherapy can help you stabilize your emotions and keep you in a positive mood. Below is a list of essential oils that you can use to alter your mood.

Essential Oils to Balance Your Mood

To reduce anger	Rose, honeysuckle, sandalwood, jasmine
To reduce depression	Patchouli, wintergreen, rosemary, basil, lavender, jasmine
To reduce a tired or dull mind	Camphor, basil, calamus, mint, eucalyptus, bay
To reduce fear and anxiety	Rosemary, lavender, sandalwood

Four Simple Ways to Create a Conscious Aromatic Environment

- Bring flowers into your home or work environment
- Add essential oils to a base oil and make a natural perfume
- Take several drops of essential oils and place them in an aromatherapy diffuser
- Create an aromatherapy spray mister

Flowers

Flowers are a treat, not only for your sense of smell but also for your sense of vision. If you grow your own flowers, you will always have a ready supply. Otherwise, a visit to a local florist once per week is a nice investment to make in your well-being.

Natural Perfume

Throw away your expensive artificial perfumes and make your own beautiful oil to rub on your body. If you are of vata nature, use almond or sesame oil as your base oil. These oils are very nourishing and are warming. If you are of pitta nature, use sunflower or coconut oil, they are cooling. If you are of kapha nature, use safflower oil, it is lighter and not as lubricating. To make a perfume, mix an equal amount of your constitutional base oil with your favorite blend of essential oils. The ratio of essential oil to base oil is different depending upon the essential oil used. Some are much stronger than others. Start with 4 drops per ounce and increase from there until you find the strength that you like. Apply a few drops to your body as desired.

Aromatherapy Diffuser

Aromatherapy diffusers are available at most health foods stores, boutiques and body and bath stores. They come in a wide variety of designs. Many use candles that are burned under a small pot that holds an ounce or two of water. Add a few drops of your essential oil blend into the water and light the candle. Soon, the room you are in will have a pleasant and balancing aroma.

Aromatherapy Spray Mister

Find a spray misting bottle at a local pharmacy or grocery store. Fill it up with water and add a few drops of your favorite essential oil or blend. Shake it well. Spray it around wherever you go. It is nice to spray the car and can also be nice to spray onto the face as a moisturizer. In the summertime, when you are outdoors and overheated, try spraying rose water onto your face. You can purchase it at the health food store or simply mix 2-3 drops of rose otto essential oil into an 8-oz misting bottle filled with water. Shake and spray.

Reflections

The use of aromatherapy is a joy. I first became interested in it when I began studying and that interest grew into growing flowers. I don't have time for extensive gardening but I do enjoy growing roses, cutting them and placing them in a nice arrangement around my house. Roses pacify pitta, purify the air and uplift the spirit. When I am hot, I carry a spray of rose water around with me and spray my face. About a year ago, I developed a blend of essential oils that I really enjoy. I apply the blend with a base oil to my body daily. Of course, with a predominantly pitta nature, I use sunflower oil as my base oil.

LESSON 11: HEALING YOUR LIFE THROUGH VISION

Color and Beauty

We are not only what we eat and smell, we are also what we see. Through our eyes, we take in a tremendous amount of information that affects our minds and emotions. These in turn affect the physiology of our bodies. If what we take in through our sense of vision is not harmonious, we will experience some level of stress and that creates disease.

Post traumatic stress disorder is an example of what can happen when the impressions taken in through the sense of vision are very disharmonious. While soldiers often come home from war with a variety of health disorders (headaches, neurological dysfunctions, etc) resulting from the things they've seen, similar symptoms are found in individuals who witness murders, rapes and other forms of violence. Disturbing images, even those that are natural, cause similar harm. Those who witness tragedies, such as fires and floods, are often left deeply scarred. Another milder example of what we see making us sick is the nausea that many people experience when seeing something disagreeable. Visual stress is very profound and affects us deeply.

If, on the other hand, we experience beautiful, peaceful impressions through our sense of vision, our minds will be more peaceful and our bodies healthier. Every impression alters the physiology of the body. Visual images, such as those of mountains, clouds, rivers and oceans, bring calm and balance to the nervous system and support healthy physiology. In such an environment, the mind is clearer and troubles seem to disappear. When used properly, visual impressions can be a tool used to support the healing process.

While the dramatic events that we witness have an obvious, profound and often immediate effect upon us, those that we see on a daily basis affect us more gradually but can be just as profound in the long term. Most of the visual impressions that we take in on a daily basis are those found in our home and at our work place. We take in the colors, we take in both the clutter and the empty spaces, we take in the images we see on the walls and we take in visual impressions of our co-workers. Though unconscious of their effect, we absorb them and they become a part of our consciousness. The impressions that we expose ourselves to on a daily basis may not be as dramatic as those witnessed on the battlefield but their impact penetrates us slowly and deeply. Like water that continuously drips onto a rock, those impressions slowly carve a groove in our consciousness. Depending upon what we look at on a daily basis, that carving can be beautiful and peaceful or quite disturbing. It is the goal of Ayurveda to become conscious of the visual environment we expose ourselves to and to begin to structure it in a manner that is supportive to our well-being.

Movies and Television

When you go out to eat, are you interested in the quality of the food at the restaurant? Does it matter to you what they serve? Of course it does. If the food is not healthy, it will give you indigestion and it can make you sick. The same is true of your choices regarding what you visually expose yourself to. Of course, by this I mean movies and television.

One of my teachers used to tell me that the mind does not know the difference between what is real and what is imagined. This is mostly true. While the intellect often discerns the difference, the emotional aspect of our consciousness does not. A happy scene in a movie causes the brain to secrete chemicals that make you happy and relaxed (dopamine, serotonin, tryptophan, phenylethylamine, anandamide). An intense scene in a movie causes the brain and adrenal glands to secrete chemicals that make you tense (epinephrine and norepinephrine). The chemicals of tension, fear and anger stimulate the sympathetic nervous system. This is that part of the nervous system that controls the "fight or flight" response. Once it is activated, the neurochemicals that are secreted circulate through your body for several hours before being deactivated.

The fight or flight response is meant to allow the body to deal effectively with threats. When a real threat is perceived, the heart rate increases to allow more blood to flow to the muscles of the body in case you need to fight or run for your life. Additional chemicals are secreted in the body that cause it to become more alert. Vision improves, strength increases and the breath is easier. These changes do not just disappear after the threat is gone. They stay with you for quite some time. Overactivation of this system has been understood to be a contributing factor in all stress-related illnesses. These illnesses include everything from arthritis and headaches to heart attacks and strokes.

If the visual impression is strong, the mind will replay it again and again and this continues to trigger the fight or flight response. It is not easy to block out a tragedy that you have witnessed. Likewise, an impactful scene in a movie may be replayed over and over again in your mind and trigger the same feelings again and again. If the scene was intense, the fight or flight mechanism is activated each time and the body functions in a continuous state of sympathetic stress.

Ask yourself what you are taking into your mind and consciousness when you are watching television or a movie. Are you watching horror movies, suspense and action films? These are sure to activate your sympathetic nervous system. At times, they can be fun, isn't that why we watch them? A part of us likes the adrenaline rush of sympathetic stimulation. But, at other times, they can be disturbing. What is the value in watching a movie about child abduction? What is the value of witnessing a murder? Violence in movies and on television is quite extensive and people lap it up just like white flour, sugar and deep-fried foods. It is a quick thrill, but with a price to our physical and mental health.

On the other hand, lighter films and comedies have been shown to have value in supporting the healing process. They encourage us to take life less seriously. Comedies also cause the brain to secrete chemicals. They could be called laughter chemicals. These chemicals relax the body and support the healing process. This was brought to the public eye in the popular book at the time by Norman Cousins called "Anatomy of an Illness".

Next time you rent a movie, ask yourself this. If this movie were a food, what food would it be? Are you about to consume fast-food junk, cookies and ice-cream or a bowl of organic brown rice and vegetables? Sometimes you may like to have dessert, but it is not healthy if you take it too often. Movies and television are the same way. An occasional adrenaline rush is not a problem for most people, but if you are highly sensitive or if it becomes the bulk of your visual diet, you will cause yourself harm. Some of the most intense movies are like food poisoning. It's just not a good idea to consume them at all.

Color and Healing

Color is a vibrational energy that enters the eye and goes directly to the brain affecting us physically and emotionally. This can be easily observed. Do you feel more powerful or confident when you wear bright red clothing or ride in a bright red car? Red is powerful and can intimidate others. This is the idea behind the red power tie used in business by men and the red suit worn by women. And how do you feel when you wear black or drive a black car. Do you feel mysterious or on the edge of being dangerous? When you see someone dressed in black, are they easy to approach? Probably not, unless you are also powerful and supremely confident. The color black separates a person from their environment allowing in only the most powerful forces. Indeed, color affects us very deeply.

While the effect of color is easy to observe on the mind, color also affects the body. New-born babies experiencing jaundice (yellowing of the skin due to excess bilirubin in the blood) are routinely treated with blue lights. The color blue alters the physiology of the body, making it possible to break down excess bilirubin into a form that can be easily excreted from the body. In this case, the color blue saves the life of the child. The effects of color on the body are only partially understood, but there can be no doubt that every color impression has a physiological effect.

From an ayurvedic perspective, all color contains some of the fire element. The fire element provides the light or luster through which all color travels. However, each color also has its own unique combination of the five elements and thus has its own unique set of qualities. Understanding the qualities of color allows you to consciously use color to support your healing process.

Fire provides the light that allows us to see color. As a color becomes richer, there is more fire in the color. At first, the influence of fire and its heat is minimal, but as the color becomes more and more intense, it becomes hotter and hotter. This is true for any color. Thus, intensely bright colors, as one might see in a laser light show, are always heating, increase the pitta dosha and are stimulating to the mind. Softer colors like pastels, on the other hand, are generally cooler and more calming than their brighter counterparts.

Red (K-PV+)

Best Use: Aphrodisiac

The color red is made up primarily of fire and air. These are the same elements that make up the pungent taste and, if red had a taste, it would be pungent. The qualities of the color red include being hot, sharp, light, mobile and dry. The brighter the color, the more fire in it. Darker reds, like magenta, have some secondary earth and are slightly cooler and heavier.

The color red is the hottest color, is very exciting and can be intense. It is an aphrodisiac, stimulating the senses more than any other color. Red lipstick, red nails and red underwear are very provocative. Red is powerful and makes a statement that you are to be noticed and reckoned with. If the color is overused, however, it expresses narcissism and a strong ego.

The color red, being hot, increases pitta dosha. I do not recommend that those with a pitta constitution or imbalance use much of the color red. While a red accent here and there will not greatly increase pitta dosha, too much red in the environment will and it will result in overheating the mind and the body. Excessive use of the color red increases judgment, passion, anger, and intensity, and makes a person more critical. In the body, this can result in an overheated liver, increased inflammation, red eyes and red skin rashes.

The color red being light, dry and mobile increases the vata dosha. Thus, I don't recommend that those with a vata nature or imbalance use much of it either. Again, accents here and there are fine and won't cause much imbalance.

For much of the same reason that the color red aggravates the vata and pitta doshas, it brings balance to kapha dosha and it is the kapha dosha that thrives the most in a red environment. The color red provides many qualities that balance out kapha's tendencies, which are heavy, moist and stable, as well as cool. Still, if the color red is too bright or intense, it will eventually cause agitation, even to kapha.

How much of the color red you can handle in a healthy manner depends a lot on your level of internal strength, which is called ojas. The weaker or less stable you are, the less you should use it. If your internal strength is high and your mind is stable, you can use it with little concern.

Orange (VK-P+)

Best Use: Increases Joy

The color orange is made up of several elements, primarily fire and air. But, unlike the color red, it also contains some earth and water. If you could taste the color orange, it would be rather sour. Orange has many of the qualities of the sour taste. It is warm, light (but not too light), dry (but not too dry), mobile and sharp. The brighter the color, the greater the amount of fire and the hotter and drier it becomes.

Like the color red, orange is exciting but not nearly as intense. It is uplifting, joyful and stimulating to the mind. It helps to lift depression and stimulate the intellect. In the body, it improves digestion and, if it is bright, it stimulates sexual energy.

Being warm, orange increases pitta dosha and can overheat the body and mind if it is used in excess by a person with a pitta nature or imbalance. This is especially true if the color is very bright. However, pastel oranges are somewhat cooler and safer to use. If you have a pitta imbalance, I would not recommend using much orange at all. However, if you have a pitta nature and are in reasonably good balance, you can use orange with little concern. Just try to avoid excessively bright shades.

If you have a vata constitution, you will benefit from some orange in your environment. It will help you to create a feeling of warmth while also being uplifting. If there is a vata imbalance or weakness present, it is best to stick to earthier shades of orange. These are still warm but are less stimulating.

Those with a kapha nature can enjoy bright shades of orange. These are warm, stimulating and uplifting while being less agitating than the color red.

Yellow (VK-P+)

Best Use: Increases Enthusiasm

The color yellow is made up of fire and ether along with a little water. The influence of fire makes the color warming. The influence of ether brings in a lighter and more expansive quality than either red or orange. In addition to being light and warm, it stimulates mobility and activity. When the sun is shining, we all want to go out and play. There is enough of the water element present to prevent the color from being drying but it is not very moist. Lacking in earth, yellow is not very heavy or stable and thus an excessive use of yellow can become ungrounding. Bright, intense yellow color is quite sharp and hard, whereas softer yellows are neither very sharp nor dull.

The color of sunshine, yellow is the most uplifting of all colors and increases one's joy and enthusiasm for life. It is a natural antidote to depression; it stimulates the intellect and increases perception.

Being warm, yellow increases pitta dosha and thus should not be overused.

This is not to mean that a person with a pitta nature should avoid it, rather it should be used in moderation. However, if pitta dosha is out of balance and there is excessive intensity and focus on accomplishment, then the color yellow should only be used minimally.

Kapha and vata doshas benefit from having more yellow in their environment as the color is warming. A person with a vata nature, however, should use some caution and not overexpose themselves or use shades of yellow that are too bright. Containing ether, excessive use of the color yellow will increase vata dosha and can contribute to imbalances. This is seen in parts of the world where the sun shines for very long hours. Sleep is difficult and, after several weeks, vata dosha rises and there is anxiety and agitation. These same qualities are the reason why the yellow color is so beneficial to kapha dosha. A person with a kapha nature has enough earth (grounding) in their nature to be only modestly affected. Imbalance does not readily occur. Rather, the extra motivation and inspiration is welcome. Thus, the color yellow should be used often in a person with a kapha nature or imbalance.

Those with a vata nature and imbalance benefit from softer yellow influences, which are less agitating, and shades of yellow with some earth in it such as gold. Those with a kapha nature or imbalance benefit from brighter shades as well as greater use of yellow color.

Gold (VPK-)

Best Use: Increases Clarity

The color gold is made up primarily of fire, water and earth but also has a little ether and air. While fire is a predominant element in the color, the heating quality of the color is tempered by influences of the other elements. Because of the influence of earth and water, gold is the heaviest of the warming colors and the most nourishing. Gold is warm, slightly moist, heavy and stabilizing.

In the mind, the color gold promotes stability and can be beneficial as part of a complete plan to manage anxiety and bi-polar tendencies. It accomplishes this without any sedative side effects. In fact, the color gold is energizing in a manner that promotes endurance rather than a quick high. It uplifts the spirit and helps to transform consciousness, as it promotes greater awareness. In the body, the color gold supports all immune functions. It helps prevent disease and is useful in the management of autoimmune disease.

For a person of vata nature, gold is protective against excessive mobility and dryness. It brings needed stability and endurance against stress. Thus, a person with a vata nature or imbalance should use this color liberally. Wearing gold jewelry is beneficial for similar reasons.

For a person with a pitta nature, gold ignites the clarity of the mind while also providing stability. Ordinarily, this illuminating quality could be too hot for a person who already has enough fire in their nature. However, in balance with water, the effect of the light given off by gold's fire creates clarity without creating intensity. This makes the use of the color gold safe for a person with a pitta nature or imbalance.

For a person with a kapha nature, the fire inherent in gold provides warmth, clarity and some stimulation. This is tempered by the stabilizing qualities of the earth in gold. Thus, gold has a neutral effect on a person with a kapha nature or imbalance.

As you can see from the description, gold is neither very balancing nor very disturbing to any one dosha. It is safe to use by everyone. This makes gold a tridoshic color.

Green: VK-P+ (only in excess)
Best Use: Brings Balance

The color green is made up of fire, water and earth in relatively equal proportions, making the qualities of the color mild and generally fine for all constitutions. It is slightly warming while being neutral in most of qualities. Green is a balancing color that has a tendency to neutralize imbalances in either direction. For instance, the use of green supports weight loss in a person who is heavy and weight gain in a person who is too light. Unlike gold, its actions are not as long lasting. It does not strongly support the immune system or aid the transformation of consciousness. Still, it is quite balanced for all three doshas. Only pitta is increased when it is used in excess. In the body, the color green stimulates the liver and gallbladder promoting bile secretions. The use of green should be minimized if there is liver inflammation.

For the person with a vata nature or imbalance, green offers stability as well as some warmth and moisture. The color green is helpful in eliminating the swings of excesses and deficiencies. This makes it useful for mood swings, bi-polar tendencies and weight that tends to yo-yo - going up and down. The color green is not as grounding as brown or as strength building as gold. However, it works well with both of these colors supporting their basic actions.

For the person with a pitta nature, the color green can help to improve the circulation of energy in the liver. Green is the color of bile, a digestive fluid that is produced in the liver and stored in the gallbladder. In small and moderate amounts, the color green disperses heat and cleanses the liver. However, in excess, its inherent warm quality results in a buildup of heat. This is like a spice that is a little warming. In general, the color green is fine for pitta dosha unless there is a strong imbalance. When pitta dosha is very aggravated, the color green should only be used as an accent.

For the person with a kapha nature or imbalance, the color green removes stagnation that is sometimes found in the liver and gallbladder. By improving bile flow, the digestion of fats is improved and there is less heaviness in the abdomen. While the color green is stabilizing, a quality that a person with a kapha nature should generally avoid, its unique effect upon liver stagnation makes it an acceptable color to help keep the kapha dosha in balance.

Blue (PK-V+)

Best Use: Purification

The color blue is made up of air and ether, the same elements that make up the vata dosha. If the color blue were a taste, it would be bitter, as the bitter taste is composed of the same elements. It is the coldest of the colors, very light, very dry, mobile and sharp.

The color blue antidotes the critical mind and the anger it generates. Blue is expansive and opens up the mind to possibilities while reducing attachment to ideas. In the body, the color blue is purifying in the manner that an antibiotic is purifying. It cools and supports the purification of the blood. While not strong enough to be relied upon as an antibiotic, it can be used to support this action in the body. The cooling nature of the color blue is also beneficial in the management of fever. As noted earlier, the color blue is beneficial in the treatment of infantile jaundice.

For the person with a vata nature, the color blue should be used with caution. It will increase all of the qualities associated with the vata dosha and even moderate use can increase anxiety, tics, tremors and pain in the body. If there is weight loss, the use of the blue color works against stabilization and further weight loss is possible. This is true for both dark blues and light pastel blues. The pastel color is even more expansive and un-grounding, while the darker blues are colder and drier.

For the person with a pitta nature or imbalance, the color blue is wonderful. It cools the mind, decreases anger, counters inflammation and reduces any buildup of excess heat in the liver or the blood. Thus, it is useful for infections of all kinds and inflammation anywhere in the body. Its regular use helps to prevent pitta imbalances as well.

For the person with a kapha nature or imbalance, the color blue is beneficial for its dry, light and mobile qualities. Thus, it helps to reduce mucous in the body, supports weight loss and helps to reduce stagnation. It helps to clear and sharpen the mind and reduce lethargy and sluggishness.

White (PK-V+)

Best Use: Promotes Meditation and Spiritual Awareness

The color white is made up of ether. Ether is known more for its lack of qualities than for any particular quality. Thus, the color white is sometimes considered to be lack of color. Lacking fire, the color white is cold. Lacking water, it is dry. Lacking earth, it is light, subtle and unstable. Lacking air, it has no propulsive action. However, it does have a natural, effortless, expansive and flowing nature.

In the mind, the color white increases the flow of creative ideas. It is also purifying and removes excesses of other qualities, such as the heat of fire and the dullness of earth. White is useful for reducing the ignorance that breeds hatred, fear and over-attachment. Because of its light qualities, it is not very grounding and so those prone to daydreaming—having their head in the clouds, should use this color as an accent only. Too much use of the color white can also increase anxiety. At the level of consciousness, the color white creates clarity and removes the obstructions that separate our individual awareness from divine awareness. Thus, white is useful for meditation and is considered to be the most spiritual of all colors, as it supports spiritual growth and inner peace. In the body, the color white is purifying and helps to remove toxins. It also supports weight loss.

For the person with a vata nature or imbalance, the color white can be too light and excessive use can lead to dizziness, feelings of being un-grounded and anxiety. Reducing the stable quality, the color white can aggravate mood swings and bi-polar tendencies. In the body, the use of the color white makes it harder to gain weight; it can increase pain and aggravate nerve disorders. Thus, the color white should be used with caution in a person with a vata imbalance. If there is a severe imbalance, it would be best to avoid it. Otherwise, it is fine to use as an accent color.

For the person with a pitta nature, the color white is very beneficial. It helps to lighten the mind and decrease seriousness. It makes a person less critical as they see life with more clarity but less judgment. In this regard, it works well with the color blue. While its subtle actions are most noticeable on the mind, they also affect the body. The color white works to prevent a buildup of excess heat in the digestive system, the liver and the blood, and in the eyes and the skin. For treating excessive heat, it is best to mix the color white with the color blue.

For the person with a kapha nature, the color white is very supportive. Being light and subtle, it helps to bring balance to the heavy, gross qualities of kapha. It can be used as part of a program to reduce weight gain, reduce mucus, increase mental clarity and sharpen the senses. If a person feels like they are stuck in a rut or melancholic, the use of the color white is the antidote, allowing for a greater flow of creative ideas and new inspiration. A person with a kapha nature can use the color white either preventively or as a part of the treatment of kapha imbalances.

Black (VPK+)
Best Use: Promotes Contemplation
The color black is the end result of mixing all colors together and hence, it contains all five elements. Earth is the most dominant element but all of the elements are well represented. When the mix is complete, its major qualities are heavy, dry, hard and cloudy. This results in a contractive nature. If black were

a taste, it would be rather astringent, as its nature is to draw energy within. Black is very powerful. It is the least subtle of the colors and has a very strong effect on the mind.

In the mind, the color black leads to introversion, contemplation and often feelings of isolation. Excessive use leads to separation from mainstream society and often to an increased desire to explore the darker side of consciousness. Those who use excessive amount of the color black often form a subculture and their social interactions become limited to those within this subculture. Examples of this occur within the Gothic and Emo subcultures where the use of black is dominant as a style of dress and makeup. We also see the use of black leather jacket by motorcycle bikers to separate themselves from non-riders. Even the black dress has a similar effect. It is worn to stand out and apart from others while creating mystery and intrigue. Not every subculture that focuses on black is the same. However, they share a fundamental similarity in that each uses the color black to separate them and explore some aspect of the "shadow", the darker, mysterious side of human nature. In those with disassociative tendencies, excessive use of the color black contributes to an inability to separate the real from the imaginary. The end result can be quite serious and lead to psychosis.

At the level of consciousness, the effect of black depends upon the spiritual development of the person using the color. In a person who is highly spiritual, having a clear mind with a deep connection to spirit, the color black acts as a barrier to the physical world and all of its temptations. This allows attention to remain internalized for deep contemplation and communion with spirit. Thus, black is the color of the monkish priest. However, in those without a deep spiritual connection, excessive use of the color black enhances the ego (the lower self). It leads to self indulgence, excesses of emotion, violence, drugs and deviant sex (intense sex with associated violence).

The color black increases all three doshas. It is too dry for vata dosha, too sharp for pitta dosha and too heavy for kapha dosha. In general, the color black should only be used with a conscious intention and without that, it is a good idea to limit its use to an accent color.

Brown (VP-K+)
Best Use: Grounding and Stability

The color brown is made up of the earth and water elements. These are the same elements that make up the kapha dosha and as such, their qualities are identical. The color brown is cool, heavy, stable, slightly dry, gross, soft, and dense. If the color brown had a taste, it would be sweet.

The color brown is nurturing and stabilizing for the body and the mind. Of all the colors, it is best for promoting strength. In the mind, it stabilizes emotions. It is grounding and helps to reduce anxiety and mood swings. It also helps control anger. Excessive use can lead to melancholy and a lack of creativity. In the body, it supports the development and growth of new tissues. It supports weight gain, muscle strength and bone growth. Excessive use can lead to stagnation and lethargy.

For the person with a vata nature or imbalance, brown is a terrific color for anchoring the mind and creating stability. The brown color is almost opposite of the vata dosha in its qualities and this is very beneficial. With somewhat of a sedative quality, the color brown reduces the effect of stress. If you need help controlling anxiety and overwhelm or preventing mood swings, brown is a very good color for you. In the body, it supports the immune system and helps to increase weight.

For the person with a pitta nature or imbalance, brown brings cooling and stabilizing qualities, inhibits excitability and prevents flare-ups of fire. This helps to prevent anger and volatile episodes. The expression of anger is due to a buildup of heat combined with mobility. Brown, while not as cold as the color blue and not as strong of an anti-inflammatory, offers a longer lasting cooling quality. It is best for long-term challenges with excess heat in the body or mind. Thus, if you are having anger management problems or chronic inflammation, brown, while working slowly, is a very good color for you.

For the person with a kapha nature or imbalance, the regular use of the brown color can lead to imbalances. Its heavy and moist nature promotes lethargy, melancholy and mucus formation in the body. It also promotes weight gain. If you are troubled with these conditions, reduce the amount of brown color that you are exposed to. Brown brings dullness to the mind and increases stubbornness. If you have a kapha nature, you should minimize your use of the color brown. If you have a kapha imbalance, it is best to avoid it or use it only as an accent.

Blended Colors

Colors can be blended to produce infinite combinations and shades. To understand the effect of color blending, it helps to know which colors make up the blend and then combine the qualities of the colors together in the proportions of the mix. However, each blend and shade is really a unique stand alone color and emits its own vibration. The most accurate understanding of the qualities of a blended color is obtained through self-observation, meditation and contemplation.

Purple (VK-P+)

Purple is a blend of red and blue with more red than blue and as such it contains more of the fire element and less earth, air and ether. It is a warm color but not hot. It is neither very light nor heavy. It is a little dry, sharp and rough.

For the person with a vata nature, the color purple provides warmth with a gentle stimulation. It is uplifting and useful for depression. Long-term, excessive use, however, does not provide the stability that a person with a vata nature needs for balance. Thus, its use should be combined with stabilizing colors, such as brown and gold.

For the person with a pitta nature or imbalance, the color purple can be a little too warming. This is especially true for brighter versions of the color. It increases the fire of perception in the mind and generates heat. This can lead to an imbalance. If you have a pitta imbalance, you should avoid excessive use of this color. However, if you have a pitta nature and are in balance, moderate use of the color purple is fine.

For the person with a kapha nature or imbalance, the use of the color purple is very balancing. It stimulates the body and mind, reduces lethargy and promotes clarity. Of the three doshas, kapha is reduced most by the color purple. Being less agitating to the mind than the color red, it is a better choice for regular use.

Violet (PK-V+)

Violet is also a blend of red and blue but with more blue than red. This makes violet a slightly cooling color and better than purple for the pitta dosha. It contains significant air and ether and less fire. It is an energizing color that removes impurities from the body and mind, thus promoting clarity. Violet promotes inspiration, as well as the energy to manifest one's dreams. In order to sustain that energy over a long period of time, however, strength and stability are needed. Violet is best for balancing the pitta and kapha doshas but can increase the vata dosha. Lavender is a lighter version of violet with more etheric qualities.

In the person with a vata nature or imbalance, violet is a little too cooling for regular use. Overuse can bring about agitation and anxiety. Though safer than the color blue, it is still too light and un-grounding to use regularly.

For the person with a pitta nature or imbalance, surrounding yourself with violet is a healthy choice. It promotes clarity without exciting the internal fire. It is safer to use than purple. It is not as cooling as the color blue, which is better for strongly reducing the fire.

For the person with a kapha nature or imbalance, the use of the color violet is a healthy choice. Being light and dry, it reduces mucus in the body. In the mind, it brings clarity, reduces lethargy, improves receptivity and promotes inspiration.

Pink (K-VP+)

Pink is a blend of red and white. The shade of pink a person is exposed to can dramatically alter its qualities. Bright or hot pink contains a lot more fire and has an effect on the body and mind that retains the exciting qualities of red while slightly reducing its intensity and drying nature. Pink is playful and less intimidating than red while still acting as a strong aphrodisiac. Pink is often the favorite color of girls, teenagers and young women because it is strongly feminine in nature while less powerful and dangerous than red. Pink consists primarily of ether and fire but also contains some air.

For the person with a vata nature or imbalance, pink is too light and stimulating. By decreasing how grounded a person feels, it promotes anxiety and nervousness. For this reason, it is best used as an accent color or for shorter durations.

For the person with a pitta nature or imbalance, the color pink is too warming. It is not as hot as red and thus not quite as overheating to the mind or body. However, it is still warming and as such, it should be used in modest amounts as an accent color. Overuse contributes to making a person more judgmental and critical. If you have a pitta nature but no significant pitta imbalance, the color pink can be used in moderation. If there is imbalance, it should be avoided.

For the person with a kapha nature, the color pink is very balancing. It is uplifting, motivating and inspirational. It helps to remove lethargy and promotes clarity. In the body, it helps to dry up mucus.

Summary: The Qualities of Color

Color	Elements	Important Qualities	Doshic Effect
Red	Fire, Air	Hot, light, mobile, dry, sharp	K-VP+
Orange	Primary: Fire, Air Secondary: Earth, Water	Warm, light, mobile	KV-P+
Yellow	Primary: Fire and Ether Secondary: Water	Warm, light, mobile	KV-P+
Green	Fire, Water, Earth	Warm, stabilizing	VK-P+ (excess)
Gold	Fire, Water, Earth	Warm, heavy, moist, stabilizing	VPK-
Blue	Air and Ether	Cold, light, dry, mobile	PK-V+
Black	All Five Elements	Cold, contractive	VK+P+ (excess)
White	Ether	Cold, light, dry	PK-V+
Brown	Water, Earth	Cold, heavy, moist, stable	VP-K+
Purple	Primary: Fire Secondary: Air, Ether, Earth	Warm, light, mobile	VK-P+
Violet	Primary: Air, Ether Secondary: Fire	Cool, light, mobile	PK-V+
Pink	Fire, Ether with scondary Air	Warm, light	K-VP+

Using Color to Heal the Doshas

Depending upon your constitution and the nature of any imbalances, certain colors will support your well-being and others will contribute to imbalances that make healing more difficult. The conscious use of color requires that you first understand the qualities inherent in color and how they affect the three doshas and then how to use color in your life.

Healing Vata Dosha with Color

Vata dosha benefits from colors that have the opposite qualities of the dosha. Thus, vata benefits from warm, moist, heavy, stable and gross qualities as well as soft, dense, dull, smooth and cloudy qualities. There is no one color that will provide vata with all of the benefits that it needs to stay in balance. Thus it is necessary to use several colors in order to bring about the maximum benefits and restore balance.

When it comes to color, the most important qualities to consider in bringing vata into balance are vata's cold and mobile qualities. These are balanced by warmth and stability. Most colors that are warming also have a mobile quality. Yellow, orange and violet are fine colors for vata but alone can create too much excitement and energy leading to greater anxiety and a loss of focus. To remedy this, it is important to also use a healthy amount of the brown and gold colors which, containing the earth element, are heavier, grounding and stabilizing. Earthy tones of orange and yellow are also better balanced than brighter and lighter tones. In general, deep, rich colors (not brighter) are the best forms of color to use to balance vata dosha. Softer pastel colors are the next best. Bright, iridescent colors are the most disturbing.

Healing Pitta Dosha with Color

Pitta dosha benefits from colors that are opposite to its natural tendencies. Since the most important factor that causes pitta to move out of balance is heat, it is the cool colors that benefit pitta the most. The blue color, being the coldest of the colors, has the quickest effect on reducing excesses of the pitta dosha. Its effect is short lived, however, because the color is so light and unstable. Brown, on the other hand, being cooling and heavy, has a greater long-term cooling effect. White is cool but also light and excessive use can aggravate weakness, if weakness is present. Violet is a cooling color bringing clarity to the mind without aggravating pitta. Gold, though a little warming, is safe for a person with a pitta nature to use as it protects a person against excesses of all qualities, including heat. The color green is fairly neutral in its action on pitta but because it can stimulate the liver, it should be avoided if there is a significant excess heat in the liver.

In general, the colors that bring balance to pitta dosha are best in their pastel form. These are softer and more calming. Deeper, richer colors are the next best. Excessively bright or iridescent colors should be avoided, as their sharpness aggravates pitta.

Healing Kapha Dosha with Color

Kapha benefits from colors that are opposite to its natural qualities. Of kapha's qualities, it is most important to reduce its heavy, moist and stable nature. These are antidoted by light, dry and mobile qualities.

The color red, being hot, light, mobile and dry, is the single most balancing color for kapha. However, if the red is too intense or if it is overly emphasized in the environment, it becomes agitating to the mind. Thus, other kapha-balancing colors should be utilized as well. White is the lightest and most expansive of the colors and creates the space for kapha to move and expand. Yellow and orange are warm, mobile and light and help motivate kapha with much less risk of irritation than red. The color blue is also beneficial for kapha even through it is cold. Blue is very light, dry and mobile and supports reducing mucus and keeping body weight in check. It can play an important role in bringing kapha into balance but should be balanced with warmer colors. The color that causes the most disturbances is brown. It is too heavy and stable.

The form of colors that is best for a person with a kapha nature or imbalance are those that are brighter and sharper. These have more fire within them. The next best are pastel colors as they are lighter. Deep, rich colors should be used with more caution as they tend to be heavier.

The Best Colors for Each Dosha

	Vata	Pitta	Kapha
Best	Orange, yellow, green, gold, brown, purple	Gold, blue, white, brown, violet	Red, orange, yellow, green, gold, blue, white, purple, violet
Use with Caution	Red, white, blue, violet	Red, orange, yellow, purple green	Brown

Summary of the Light and Heavy Colors

The following list shows the order of colors from lightest to heaviest. The lighter colors are better for purifying and expanding the mind and are particularly beneficial for balancing the kapha dosha. The heavier colors are better for nourishing the mind and are more grounding. These are particularly beneficial for balancing the vata dosha. All colors become heavier as their tone becomes deeper and richer and lighter when in their pastel tone. Only brown, black and gold can truly be said to have a heavy quality.

- White
- Blue
- Violet
- Purple
- Red
- Yellow
- Orange
- Green
- Gold
- Black
- Brown

Summary of the Cooling and Warming Colors

The following list shows the order of the colors from coolest to warmest. The colder colors are best for the pitta dosha. The warmer colors are better for vata and kapha doshas. However, the heating or cooling quality alone cannot determine the effect on the vata and kapha doshas. Other qualities such as heavy / light and mobile / stable are also important. Only blue, white, brown and violet can be truly stated to be cooling.

- Blue
- White
- Brown
- Violet
- Green
- Gold
- Yellow
- Purple
- Orange
- Red

*Black is a cool color but retains heat

Summary of the Mobile and Stable Colors

The following list shows the order of the colors from the most mobile to the most stable. Mobile colors are beneficial for creating motivation and primarily benefit kapha dosha. Stable colors help create stability in a person's body, mind and lifestyle. Only green, gold, black and brown can truly be said to increase stability.

- Blue
- Violet
- Red
- Purple
- White
- Orange
- Yellow
- Green
- Gold
- Black
- Brown

Conscious Vision - Building a Beautiful and Healthy Visual Environment

The Clothes You Wear

The clothes that you wear affect both you and the people around you. Color emits a vibration and that vibration affects every cell of the body. Thus, whether you are looking at the color or not, you are affected. If you are looking at it, you are more strongly affected.

For your own health and well-being, the color of the clothes that you wear should support reducing the dosha that is most out of balance. If there is no significant imbalance, then colors can be chosen that are the most supportive to keeping the doshas that make up your constitution from moving out of balance. This manner of using color is preventative.

Examine your wardrobe. Most people wear a few colors over and over again. What colors do you wear? Are they supportive or are they contributing to your imbalance and making it more difficult for your body to heal itself?

For most of us, our choice of clothing is based on what we think looks good and not on what is healthy and harmonious. This is like choosing a food based only on its taste and choosing the sweetest food. At a glance, making choices based on what looks good, makes sense. There are many benefits that come from looking good. But, these benefits are all based on the success of our ego in the world. They are not based on the success of our soul and its quest for enlightenment, balance and bliss. This should not be surprising. No woman chooses to wear four-inch heels because it makes them healthier and more peaceful. Rather, the choice is made because it makes them sexy, and sex sells. Sex appeal helps the ego achieve its goals. Most color choices are based on similar priorities. Unfortunately, choices made for the pursuit of ego gratification often hinder the goals of the soul. We often sacrifice well-being for the pursuit of power, status, money and pleasure.

This is not to say that you can't look good, be effective in the world and also be healthy and have a peaceful mind. You can! But it requires re-framing your ideas of what looks good. Some people love a McDonald's Big Mac hamburger and dislike vegetables. But, with a little courage and experimentation, a person can re-learn that vegetables taste good too.

What we like and dislike is easy to influence. Each of us has a natural instinctive liking for that which brings about health and well-being. If those were our only choices, our lives would be easy. Unfortunately it is not. And, once our mind latches on to something more exciting and stimulating, we tend to replace our idea of what is healthy and harmonious with what is exciting and pleasurable. We give up water for soft drinks. There lies the problem. It doesn't take long until we disregard our natural instincts and follow the path of short-term pleasure.

So, how do we make the leap? There are two ways really; all at once or a little at a time. If you have a pitta nature, you will probably want to do it all at one time. There is no right or wrong way. When you are ready, give it a try. It is fine to look good. It is fine to look great. See if you can do it with the colors that are best for you. And use the other colors as accents.

Your Home and Work Environment

Examine your home environment. What color are the walls? If they are a shade of white, what shade is it? Is it a warm shade or a cool shade? Which would be better for you? What color is the carpet? How about the couch in your living room and the chair in your office? The colors of the walls, the carpet and the place where you sit at most often have the greatest impact on your well-being. Most of the other pieces of furniture play an accessory role. Is it time to remodel? It just might be. If you're not ready to remodel, start with small changes.

Pictures on the Wall

Take a look at the pictures on the wall. While pictures are an accessory, a dramatic picture could have a significant effect on your well-being. How do you know if it is dramatic? Ask yourself if it draws a lot of attention. If it does, then it is having a strong influence on you. What colors are used in the pictures? Is it supportive to your well-being or is it supporting the imbalance? It is not only the color of the pictures that are on your wall that is important. A picture conveys other energies that you take in through your sense of vision. Is the picture peaceful or active? Is it calming or energizing? How would you describe the elemental makeup the picture?

Fire: Fire is represented in pictures through the color red, through bright images, through actual fire, through passion and through conflict. Fire in a picture is most beneficial for kapha dosha and is most disturbing to pitta dosha. Too much of it can disturb vata dosha as well.

Water: Water is represented in pictures as oceans and rivers. Pictures of romantic love or a face or scene that evokes compassion symbolize the water element. Water is beneficial for supporting vata and pitta but causes kapha to become lethargic.

Earth: Earth is represented in pictures through the color brown and also through images of the earth itself. Mountains, hills and sturdy trees express the grounding qualities of the earth. The earth is also symbolized in images of buildings. Earth is beneficial for vata and pitta doshas but causes kapha dosha to increase.

Air: Air is represented in pictures through the color blue and also through motion. Active pictures such as those of the movement of a dancer, flying birds and running animals are examples of the energy of air within a picture. Air can also be symbolized in a picture through the busyness of the picture. A scene of a busy city with lots of details to examine is another expression of the air element. Pictures with a lot of air element represented in them increase the vata dosha while bringing balance to kapha dosha. Sometimes a person with a pitta imbalance is disturbed by excessive air in pictures, as air tends to stoke their fire.

An example of a picture-game where air is predominant is the game "Finding Waldo". In this game, Waldo is hiding somewhere within a very busy scene and your job is to find him. Your attention is drawn in many directions and to many details. There is no movement in the picture but the picture and the game causes your attention to keep moving. This increases the vata dosha. Children who have a difficult time sleeping would be well advised not to play this game before bed. As vata dosha increases, sleep decreases.

Ether: Ether is represented through the color white and also in the empty space within a picture. A large picture with a small object and lots of empty space around it is a good example. Zen-based art often emphasizes the space between the objects as much as the object itself. The emptier the picture, the more space that is present and the greater the influence of the ether element. Ether is best for those with a kapha and pitta nature but can increase the vata dosha.

Chaos, Order and Clutter

Color is not the only aspect of our environment that we take in through our eyes. We also take in the object itself, how plentiful it is and how it is arranged. This in turn affects the three doshas.

How do you feel when you walk into a room that is chaotic? Does it make you feel more overwhelmed and easily confused? It usually does, and this is because the room has been strongly affected by the energy of vata. Chaos is an expression of the mobile quality. Being in a chaotic environment raises the vata dosha in your own body and mind. This can create a vata imbalance in anyone, regardless of constitution. Likewise, if a room is well organized, efficient and ergonomically designed, it easily facilitates the flow of energy and can make you feel like you can accomplish something in that room. That room supports the energy of pitta. Anyone working in that room will be more efficient. If a room is overly full with too much furniture, there may be order but there may also be obstruction to the flow of energy. Well-organized clutter is the result of a kapha imbalance and being in that room can raise your own kapha dosha, resulting in creative energy blocks.

If you have a vata nature or imbalance, the key to staying in balance is preventing chaos. This requires planning and making the time on a regular basis to stay organized. While this may not come naturally to you, it can be accomplished with conscious effort.

If you have a pitta nature or imbalance, it is important to avoid situations that trigger excessive orderliness. Stress, such as deadlines, is often the culprit.

Thus, planning to complete tasks early allows for a more relaxed approach just in case something gets in the way. As a deadline approaches, vata-type stresses often push pitta out of balance. This is a case of air stoking a fire. For example, a person of pitta nature may become more intense when they can't find their car keys. In response, they begin to excessively clean up and yell at a few people while doing it.

For a person with a kapha nature or imbalance, avoiding clutter is important, as it further hinders energy that already moves rather slowly. Setting up a simple, beautiful but sparse environment allows energy to flow freely. If there is excessive clutter around, it may be time for a garage sale or a "give away." This is where, if you can't sell your valued possessions at a garage sale, you simply give them to your friends or a neighborhood thrift store.

Important Accents

Accent your environment with beauty. Flowers and plants are the simplest and most direct way to make the space you are living in more peaceful and healing. While flowers and plants are supportive to healing in general, the colors of the flowers can be chosen according to your constitution or according to your imbalance. Flowers have the added benefit of bringing aromatherapy into your home or work environment.

If you are living in an environment that is not very pleasant for one reason or another and you do not have the resources to move to another location, create beauty in inexpensive ways. In addition to plants, damaged walls and large areas of unsightly wall space can be covered up with beautiful wall hangings. Stained and torn couches can be covered up with large bedspreads and unsightly tables can be covered with beautiful tablecloths.

The Esoteric Uses of Color for Healing Color Meditation

Color can be used for meditation and when it is, color becomes a profound medicine. Color meditations take place with the eyes open as the meditator gazes deeply into the color, becoming fully absorbed in it. Color fills the consciousness of the observer, enhancing its effects. A few minutes of color meditation can deeply affect the mind and restore balance to the doshas.

Color Meditation Instruction

Arrange a color image at eye level or in a position where you can easily gaze at it. Depending upon the size of the image, you may be just a few feet away from it or, if it is large, quite a distance away.

Sit quietly in a comfortable position. Your legs may be crossed in a yogic sitting posture or you can sit on a chair with your feet flat on the ground or crossed at the ankles. Keep your spine straight and your head forward.

Close your eyes as you bring your awareness to your breath and feel it as it moves in and out. If you have a mantra (a sound that you focus on) repeat that mantra as you sit quietly. After a few minutes, continue to focus your attention inward on your breath and mantra and then open your eyes. Gaze at the colored object. With each breath in, imagine that you are breathing in the color. With each breath out, imagine that it is circulating through your body and bathing every cell in its light. Continue for a few minutes the first time and increase the time with each practice until you are able to sit for ten minutes. Do not be concerned if the eyes water a little while performing this meditation.

Drinking Color

Many people believe that the vibration of a color can be infused into water and alter the vibration of the water itself. When the energized water is drunk, the vibration enters the body and mind, altering the vibration of each cell and bringing about healing.

There are several ways to help color vibration enter into a glass of water. One is to choose a colored glass. It is best if the glass allows some light to pass through the wall of the glass. Blue glass is pretty easy to find. Other colors are available if you look around. If you can't find the colored glass that you like, you can wrap a clear glass in colored saran wrap. One other method is to take a gemstone of the desired color and place it into the glass. Gemstones each have their own properties beyond their color so, in addition to the color therapy, additional benefits can be gained by selecting the proper stone. To select the proper gemstone consult a Vedic astrologer.

Instruction

Once you find the right colored glass, fill it with water and, if possible, cover the top of the glass. Leave the glass in sunlight or moonlight. It is important that the light be able to pass through the colored glass into the water. Light carries the color vibration into the water. The longer the glass sits in the light, the stronger the energy of the color becomes. I suggest that you let the glass sit in the light for at least three hours. If you are you trying to decrease the pitta dosha, it is best to let the glass sit outside in the moonlight, as the moon's energy is cooling. If you are trying to reduce vata or kapha dosha, it is best to let the glass sit in the sunlight, as the sun's energy is warming. The sun or moon energy adds to the vibration of the water. Drink the water one or two times each day.

Personal Reflection

I am blessed to live in a mountain community called Grass Valley in California. When I walk out my door and wherever I go, I am surrounded by pine, fir, cedar and oak trees. My visual environment is very nourishing. Still, I recall a couple of pivotal milestones in my journey toward conscious vision.

One evening, while I was in the Los Angeles / Long Beach area teaching at our Southern California center, I was feeling bored and decided to go see a movie. A movie was playing that I heard was very, very good.

The movie was *Gangs of New York* with Leonardo DiCaprio. When the movie ended I walked out of the theater and realized that I felt empty and a little off. The movie was for the most part excellent. The acting was fantastic, the writing and directing outstanding. I recall asking myself though why would I want to see that movie. The violence and intensity of the film left me with no real joy, laughter or light-heartedness. Rather, I took into my body and mind imagery that was disturbing. Of course, I am a grown man and I know the difference between fiction and reality and I wasn't deeply wounded. I was just feeling empty.

I felt like I wasted my time, got very little in return and on a subtle level, I felt assaulted. Yes, that is the best word. Having cultivated my inner peace over the years I've clearly become more sensitive, able to discern the disruption to my energy from such an experience. The movie made me feel less peaceful. Of course, the perpetrator of the assault was not the movie, it was me. I had made the choice to see the movie even though I intellectually knew that it was not likely to be high quality visual food. My intellect had failed and now I was paying a subtle price. Since then, I have rarely exposed myself to such graphically violent and intense films, preferring instead lighthearted movies, adventures and comedies.

Another pivotal experience was when my wife and I remodeled our home. We put a lot of thought into the color scheme of the walls, carpets, couches and tiles on our hearth. We redecorated with a consciousness of color that went beyond simply color combinations but rather with an eye for balance and beauty. Prior to redecorating we lived in our house for quite a few years with the color scheme the previous owner had utilized – mostly shades of light brown and tan with little contrast. The effect the old color scheme had on us could only be described as depressing our energy. It didn't inspire us or increase our joy. After living in that environment for years, we redecorated with brighter colors using a yellow-gold faux paint on one wall, orange faux on part of the ceiling in our kitchen. We also added natural sunlight through a solar tube. The walls themselves that were not faux were brighter as well having used a solid shade of light yellow. Needless to say the yellow, gold and orange theme and the increased natural light added to our inspiration and completely shifted the energy of our living experience. In order to ground the energy we used a dark raspberry chocolate carpet in the main living room, stone slate tile around the hearth and stone porcelain tile with a deep orange stone finish in the kitchen. The couches we chose were a gentle green in the main living room picking up the color in the slate and dark green in the formal living area. The overall energy of the home now is balancing for vata dosha, slightly increasing to pitta dosha (I have to keep pitta in balance in other ways) and balancing to kapha dosha. In other words, it doesn't depress us at all anymore; it's a little warming, uplifting and is certainly joyful and inspiring. I now look forward to coming home every day.

LESSON 12: HEALING YOUR LIFE THROUGH SOUND

*I walk along the river
listening to its voice
reminding me that we are one.*

If you are what you eat, and you are what you smell, and you are what you see, then it is not surprising that you are also what you hear! Through our ears, we take in the sounds of our environment. These sounds can either be harmonious or disharmonious. Sound affects the physiology of the body. Harmonious sounds support the healing process while disharmonious sounds are stressful and contribute to disease.

It may be hard to imagine that sound can affect us so deeply, but here is an example. If you live near a construction zone and you are listening to the sounds of a jack hammer, you will soon develop signs of stress. Headaches and stomachaches are very common. This stress can even lead to ulcers. In fact, every system of your body reacts negatively to auditory stress.

It is not just the obviously obnoxious noises that cause stress and disease. Any sound that annoys us will trigger a stress reaction. This can include a baby crying on an airplane or the harsh words of someone who yells at you. How do you feel when you are called a name or are verbally insulted? Words trigger feelings and these feelings contribute to disease.

Just as some sounds cause our bodies to react in a negative manner, other sounds activate the healing process of our bodies. Most people are soothed by the sound of the ocean or the flowing waters in a river. A gentle wind moving through the trees is also generally healing. While the sounds of nature support our nervous and immune systems, so too do certain words.

How do you feel when you are complimented? If you are told you look nice, the biochemistry of your body actually adjusts in ways that make you feel good. Other healing changes occur when you hear the words, "I love you." Words that make you feel good enhance the ability of the immune system to keep your body healthy.

While the details of the biochemistry behind how our thoughts and emotions affect our immune system are still sketchy, one of the key players is believed to be a class of proteins called Interleukins. Interleukins are produced by many types of cells in the body but particularly by the white blood cells. As a group, they can be called the regulators of the immune system. Individually, they have many effects and participate in fighting off microbial diseases and cancer. One theory is that certain Interleukins are produced in greater quantity when we are excited about life. If this is true, then when you are sick, surround yourself with people who help you to feel good about yourself.

The ayurvedic art of understanding the effects of sound is even more subtle and detailed. Knowledge of this art brings the world of sound under conscious control. A word is not just a word, it is a bundle of energy which, when used properly, contributes to the healing process, and when used inappropriately, contributes to disease.

The Power of a Word

What is a word? A word is a package of energy sent from the lips of one person to the ears of another. The package is formed in the mind, translated into a word and launched by the lips. It travels through the air and enters the ear of another person penetrating their mind and consciousness. Once it does, it alters the receiver's physiology. It is a vibration whose impact goes beyond the simple meaning of the word.

It has been observed and there is some evidence that the sound environment of a plant affects its growth and health. If you talk nicely to your plants, they seem to grow better. Do plants understand words? Of course not; but they do seem to receive something. A word has its own energy. This energy is then altered by the tone and the intention in which it is spoken. The phrase, "I love you" may be one of the most powerful phrases in the English language. It evokes a deep feeling. These feelings are biochemical responses which then affect our health and well-being.

A doctor by the name of Masaru Emoto wrote a controversial book called Messages in Water. In summary, Dr. Emoto found that upon freezing water, the crystals that formed took shape based upon the energetic surroundings of the water. Factors such as words and intention appeared to affect the formation of the crystals. When harmonious intentions and words were present, the crystals that formed were beautiful. When disharmonious intentions and words were used, the crystals that emerged were deformed. This research has been used to demonstrate the power of subtle energies such as words and intention on the well-being of water. Since human beings are composed of 98% water, these same subtle energies must also affect us. It is interesting to note that Dr. Emoto found that the effect of words on water occurred regardless of whether the word was spoken, thought or just written down and placed upon a glass of water. This supposedly demonstrates that a word has its own energy outside of the context of its sound vibration, understood meaning or the intention of the person speaking the word.

If this is true, then the following explanation may help explain it. There is a saying in the study of architecture, anatomy and evolution: "Form follows function." This means that the form a structure takes depends upon the function that part is intended to play. Need precedes the actions that create the form. Taking this just a small step further into the realm of linguistics, the word is the form. The energy is the feeling that forms the word. Philosophically, this means that human beings created language to give form to the energy (feelings) they experienced and needed to communicate. This would be true regardless of the language. Thus, the word is the carrier of the energy. This energy is perceived by every living cell – plant or animal. Thus, the final energetic impact of a communication is based on the energy inherent in the words used.

Dr. Emoto's work is considered controversial. Whether you believe it or not, it should make you consider the words you use and the intention behind your words. It should also make you consider the words and intentions that are coming toward you. The verbal environment we place ourselves in is largely under our control. We have choices about whom we associate with. While some people chose to remain in verbally abusive environments, this can not be said to be healthy. On the other hand surrounding ourselves with a positive auditory environment supports the healing process.

If you are sick and trying to get well, surround yourself with positive, supportive, compassionate and loving people who speak similarly. Avoid people who are negative, critical, angry or ridden with anxiety.

The Total Energetic Impact of Communication

The exact nature of the effect any particular communication has on the receiver is complicated. The neurobiology of sound reception really hasn't been studied at this level. The major factors of importance to be studied are the words themselves, how they are spoken and the perception of the person receiving the communication. Each of these factors can be further broken down. How a word is spoken includes regional accents, the tone of voice it is spoken in, and inflections that are used. It also includes the expressed meaning and the expressed sincerity. These last two factors are the intention with which the word is spoken. Perception can be broken down into perceived meaning and perceived sincerity, There may even be more factors but it is clear that the study of the impact of a word is quite complex.

From a mathematical perspective, the total energetic effect impact of a communication depends upon each of these factors. An equation to summarize the effect would be:

TEI = W + A + I +T + EM+ ES +PM + PS

TEI =Total Energetic Impact

W = Word

A= Accent

T = Tone

EM: Expressed Meaning

ES: Expressed Sincerity

I= Inflection

PM = Perceived Meaning

PS = Perceived Sincerity

Here is an example for the purpose of demonstrating the factors:

A person says, "you are bad." Bad has a meaning that is negative. Dr. Emoto's work would suggest that the word itself, outside of the context of implied meaning, tone and so on, has a negative effect on the water molecules of the body. Yet, it would be inconceivable that the tone in which it is spoken and the expressed meaning would not alter the impact of the word in some way. If someone says to a child, "you are bad", after the child fails to follow directions, a different response will be evoked in the child if the words are spoken calmly or in a strong tone of voice. Likewise, in a completely different context, when a friend says, "you are bad", the inflection used may indicate to the perceiver that the statement is meant in jest or fun. This produces a completely different response in the receiver. This response has a different biochemical basis. Finally, the same statement, "you are bad", can be taken within some contexts to have the completely opposite meaning. It can be a compliment. Upon hearing the statement, the receiver responds positively. Each experience of the phrase must create a unique neuro-biochemical response.

If all of this seems complicated, well, it is and it isn't. While researchers will break down the different components of sound and communication into microscopic parts, Ayurveda is concerned only with the collective end result. What effect does a word or a communication have on the doshas? The answer lies in the ten pairs of opposite qualities.

A word, sentence or phrase is like a bus. Inside of the bus are the ten pairs of opposite qualities. When the bus enters the ear of the receiver, the qualities get off the bus and join with the body, mind and consciousness of the recipient. What is healing depends upon the nature of the receiver, the nature of any imbalances present and the nature of the communication.

The Qualities of Communication

Hot / Cold: Hot communication may be angry, passionate, seductive or intense. The communication often expresses judgments. Cold communication may be calm, dispassionate, aloof or distant. Hot communication increases pitta dosha. Cold communication dramatically increases vata dosha and to a lesser extent kapha dosha as well.

Moist / Dry: Moist communication is caring, compassionate or emotional in a sweet way. An example is a person who expresses empathy in a conversation. Dry communication is to the point, lacking in sweetness or affect. Moist communication increases kapha dosha. Dry communication increases vata dosha. Pitta being only slightly moist is not greatly affected by this aspect of communication.

Heavy / Light: Heavy communication is serious, deep and also sincere. Light communication is more superficial, less serious and may be insincere. Most humor is light. Politics is heavy. Light communication increases vata dosha. Heavy communication increases kapha dosha. As pitta dosha is not very heavy or light, this quality alone does not have a great affect on pitta dosha.

Mobile / Stable: Mobile communication is fast and changes direction often. This occurs when a person speaks quickly or when the topic of conversation shifts around quite a bit. Stable communication occurs slowly and the topic does not shift very often. Mobile communication increases vata dosha. Stable communication increases kapha dosha.

Sharp / Dull: Sharp communication is to the point. It also has an edge to it that often makes other people uncomfortable. Dull communication is bland, lacking in clarity and focus. Sharp communication increases vata and pitta doshas. Dull communication increases kapha dosha.

Smooth / Rough: Smooth communication occurs in a pleasant, captivating and melodious tone of voice. The words flow effortlessly and bring about calm. It is music to the ears. Rough communication occurs in a fractured, choppy and often grating manner. The effect brings irritation. Smooth communication increases kapha dosha while rough communication increases vata and pitta doshas.

Gross / Subtle: Gross communication is obvious and can not be mistaken. What you hear is what you get. Gross communication expresses the facts and deals with subjects that can be easily experienced. Subtle communication has many layers to it and is often more esoteric. Poetry is subtle. So is scripture. The meaning of subtle communication may take a while to unfold inside the listener. Gross communication increases kapha dosha. Subtle communication increases vata and pitta doshas.

Cloudy / Clear: Cloudy communication is more difficult to understand. The meaning of the communication appears hidden as if in fog or mud. Clear communication comes from a place of clarity regarding the subject. It is easier to understand, especially if the words are carefully chosen. Cloudy communication increases kapha dosha. Clear communication increases vata and pitta doshas.

Soft / Hard: Soft communication is gentle, considerate, kind and unobtrusive. Hard communication hits you over the head. It lacks in consideration, feels intrusive and does not consider the listener. Soft communication increases kapha dosha. Hard communication increases vata dosha and, to a lesser extent, pitta dosha.

Dense / Flowing: Dense communication is often complex and contains many tightly packed layers of information. It takes a long time to decipher and understand. I have been to more than a few scientific lectures where the information conveyed was so dense, I had to sit with it for several hours or even days before I fully understood it. Flowing communication on the other hand is less packed and less grounded in the present moment. It is expansive and carries the listener into subtler realms of understanding. Dense communication increases kapha dosha. Flowing communication increases vata and pitta doshas.

Communication and the Vata Dosha

A person with a vata imbalance communicates in a manner that has vata-aggravating tendencies. A person with a vata imbalance tends to speak without much passion (cold) and, speaks quickly, possibly with agitation or frequent changes of subject (mobile). Communication lacks deep concern or compassion (dry) and does not consider the listener (hard). It is rather superficial (light), grating (rough), and irritating (sharp). It carries you along, much like a story (flowing) that is told indirectly (subtle) but eventually leads to understanding (clear) if the listener follows along. This communication style is typical of an imbalance but there is a tendency to communicate in this manner in anyone who has a large amount of vata dosha in his or her constitution. Being in the presence of this style of communication causes vata dosha to rise in the listener.

If you have a vata nature or imbalance you can restore balance if you consciously communicate in a style that antidotes your tendencies. Likewise, you will experience more healing if others communicate to you similarly. For you, a balancing and healing style of communication is friendly (warm), caring and compassionate (moist), sincere (heavy) and steady (stable). It is kind (soft), pleasant (smooth) and has no edge (dull). While you are out of balance, avoid esoteric topics and try to remain grounded in the present moment (dense). This type of communication will nourish you and support your healing process.

If you have a vata imbalance, surround yourself with people who communicate with loving kindness. If you are in balance, communicate in a conscious manner, respectful of your own tendencies.

Communication and the Pitta Dosha

A person with a pitta nature or imbalance uses words that include a lot of judgment and their tone is often passionate and righteous (hot). Communication is very logical, easy to understand (clear) and to the point (sharp). More often than not, the fiery heat of pitta overwhelms the small amount of water in the dosha. This leads to dryness and hardness. As a result, communication often lacks compassion (dry) and attitudes become rigid (hard) over time. Tone and inflections become aggressive (rough). Strong judgments lead to a deeper exploration of issues. This is necessary for developing pathways of logic. As a result, conversations go deeper (heavy) than in those with a vata imbalance.

When out of balance, a person with a pitta nature communicates in absolutes and this provokes other people with pitta imbalances. As a result, arguments are quite common (unstable). This communication style is typical of an imbalance but there is a tendency to communicate in this manner in most people who have a large amount of pitta dosha in their constitution. Being in the presence of this style of communication will cause your pitta to rise. This is not so bad if you are healthy and you have a vata or kapha nature. However, if you are exhausted or your pitta dosha is out of balance, being in the presence of this type of communication is not supportive to your well-being. It ignites your own fire. Two people with pitta imbalances can really get into heated debate! When a person with a healthy pitta nature confronts a person with an unhealthy pitta nature, it is best to just walk away, smile inside and know that you could be that person if you get out of balance yourself.

Conscious communication is the key to bringing balance back to the person with a pitta disturbance. Communication that is less passionate and intense (cool) and more compassionate (moist) controls the fire. It is also helpful when the voice is pleasant (smooth) and the words chosen are kind (soft). Swami Sivananda of Rishikesh said that the Yogi should speak the truth but do so with sweetness. Sometimes the person with a pitta imbalance forgets that last part. Without sweetness, the truth, like sword, is too sharp and can cause harm. Sweetness is cool, moist, soft, dull and smooth. These are all qualities that balance and bring healing to pitta dosha.

If you have a pitta imbalance, avoid being in communication with other people who have a pitta imbalance. When you are back in balance, communicate in a conscious manner respectful of your tendencies.

Communication and the Kapha Dosha
A person with a kapha imbalance communicates in a quiet (soft), slow (stable) and rather uninspiring (heavy) manner. There may be a lot of intended meaning in their communication (dense) but it is rarely direct and to the point (dull). Thus, it is difficult to understand (cloudy). Their tone of voice is pleasant (smooth). Lacking in passion (cold), the communication style is not very motivating and it is not very critical. The words used are most often kind (soft) and they easily express compassion and empathy (moist). The here and now (gross) is the subject of their communication. Esoteric conversation is rarely initiated.

Conscious communication means surrounding yourself with people who will communicate with you in a manner that creates balance. When balance is achieved, then it is your responsibility to communicate in a manner respectful of your tendencies. This helps to prevent future imbalances.

Communication that is passionate (hot), to the point (sharp), not very complex (flowing) and easy to understand (clear) helps to create motivation and decreases lethargy. An animated delivery (mobile) that is inspired (light and subtle) also helps to move the stagnated energy. It takes a lot of energy to overcome stagnation.

Summarizing the Effect of Words and Communication

Since words are energy and we are all affected by what we hear, it only makes sense that we benefit from becoming conscious of the words we speak and those that we expose ourselves to. What type of word environment do you find yourself in? Are those around you speaking in a manner that supports your healing? Or are those around you contributing to your illness, either through negativity or ignorance? Mean-spirited, destructive communication is rarely healing. If your auditory environment is unsuited to your dosha, you will suffer on some level. Repeated exposure to any extreme communication eventually damages the mind and body of the receiver. Being in the line of fire of extreme vata communication creates anxiety in the listener. Being in the line of fire of extreme pitta communication (hateful, severely judgmental) creates anger in the listener. Being in the line of fire of extreme kapha communication (unmotivated) eventually creates lethargy and depression in the listener.

Each of us has the power of choice in our lives. If we want to be healthy, we must use that power to control our environment. No one needs to be a victim of ongoing verbal abuse. As consciousness evolves around our auditory environment, it becomes time to choose the people that we surround ourselves with. This is not easy and it can mean letting go of old friends, leaving a relationship, or changing jobs. The question is, is your well-being worth it?

Music and Healing

In addition to the people you surround yourself with there is also the musical lyrics you expose yourself to. Listen closely: Are the lyrics expressing an energy that will support your well-being and the person you want to be, or are you choosing music with lyrics that keep you bound to old thoughts and feelings that no longer serve you?

The effect of music on health is also poorly understood but this does not make it unimportant. Music is making up more and more of our auditory environment. With the invention of the I-pod came the personal soundscape. It is without question that music affects the brain and impacts neurological functioning. Music provokes feeling and emotion and this is the reason it is so popular. Emotion is biochemical and these biochemicals directly affect every system of our body, including our immune systems. Music has an impact on physiological function and dysfunction in the body. Knowledge of the effect of music can help you create a healing environment.

Can music be used as medicine? According to Ayurveda, it can. While Western science understands music in terms of pitch, tone, frequency, harmonics, time signatures and rhythm, ayurvedic medicine understands it in terms of the ten pairs of opposite qualities. Some music is mobile. The faster the beat, the more mobile its quality and the more energizing its effect. This is better for bringing balance to kapha dosha but can lead to imbalance in vata and pitta doshas. Other music moves slowly and is calming or stable. This is better for individuals with a vata or pitta nature but may lead to an imbalance in those with a kapha nature or imbalance. Music can be further understood in terms of the other nine pairs of opposite qualities.

The Effects of Various Genres of Music on the Three Doshas

While the following conclusions are based upon the overall qualities of the genre, within any genre there is variation and that needs to be considered and respected. Absolute statements cannot be made about any genre of music but important conclusions can still be drawn. If you often listen to a form of music that is not ideal for you, it may be helpful to reduce it. This is especially important if you are sick. However, if your body and mind are healthy, moderation may be more appropriate.

Rock and Roll: K-VP+

Rock and role music contains a lot of fire and air. As such, it is generally hot and mobile. It is passionate and moves the body and the mind. This is best for those with a kapha nature or imbalance.

Hard Rock / Heavy Metal / Death Metal: K-VP+

Hard rock, heavy and death metal genres contain a predominance of the air, fire and earth elements. As such, the genre is mobile, hot and heavy respectively. This music can aggravate any of the doshas but is most imbalancing to vata and pitta doshas and most beneficial to kapha dosha. If the mind is very dull, this type of music and stimulation can be balancing.

Jazz: KP-V+

Jazz is dominated by the air element though other elements mix in with it. It is mobile and generally neither too hot nor too cool. There are many sub genres of jazz and each has slightly different qualities. The improvisational (mobile) nature of jazz, as well as the occasional discordance (light and purifying) aggravates the vata dosha.

Smooth Jazz: VP-K+

Smooth jazz contains more water and ether than classical jazz. As the genre implies, it is smoother and softer. It is gentler and less mobile. It is better for those with a vata nature, fine for pitta but may not be motivating enough to bring balance to kapha dosha.

New Age: P-VK+ (ex)

New-age music includes meditation music, gentle quiet guitar or piano music, and nature's sounds. It contains more ether than other forms of music. These sounds are light, cooling, soft and smooth. They calm the body and the mind and are best for those with a pitta nature. Those with a vata nature are also soothed by this music and it can help to calm the nerves. However, an excessive amount of this music is too light and ungrounding. For those with a kapha nature, this music provides little motivation though it can create inspiration.

Rap: K-VP+

Rap music if filled with fire and air and tends to be hot and mobile. This makes it best for those with a kapha nature and aggravating for those with a vata or pitta nature. When the lyrics are positive, rap music can help create a supportive environment for healing stagnation.

Reggae: PK- V+ (ex)

Reggae music is mobile and flowing. It is dominant in the air and water elements. The watery nature of the rhythm moves the body and mind like a swell in the ocean. It is not as mobile as most rock and roll music and is therefore less agitating to vata. Still, if a person with a vata nature is out of balance, any excess motion should be avoided. For those with a pitta nature, the cooling pleasure generated by the music is healing. For those with a kapha nature, the mobile quality is supportive and motivating.

There are many more styles of music of course. World music as a genre has a varying quality depending upon the part of the world the music originates from. Folk music is generally musically calmer and better for vata dosha. However the lyrics may be quite fiery and passionate. The blues tend to be more earthy and heavier. The blues can ground vata and pitta dosha but is too heavy for kapha dosha.

Within any style of music there are always exceptions. It is best to begin to listen for the qualities within music and then to choose the music that best suits your nature.

Mantra and Healing

A mantra is a sacred sound. Mantras have been used for thousands of years as a tool for affecting consciousness. The ancient rishis (mystical seers) of India were well aware of the effect that sound has on the mind and the deeper aspects of our being. They developed a science for using mantra to aid the healing process, clear the mind of obstacles, awaken awareness, and bring about enlightenment.

Some mantras are single words. Others are sentences or statements. They are powerful sounds that, when repeated, are intended to either etch a positive groove within one's consciousness or heal a negative groove that already exists. Each groove is a tendency, which in Sanskrit is called a "samskara." Each samskara distorts our experiences of the world. As such we never perceive pure truth; we only perceive that which is filtered through the clouds of our consciousness.

The science of using mantra is quite well developed and is called "mantra yoga." Another form of sound yoga is called "nada yoga" which focuses more on internal sounds or vibrations. Some mantras are single syllables or seed sounds called bija mantras. Others are several words or sentences that express an aspect of nature or the divine. Each mantra combines sound with a focal point of concentration. For instance, when chanting a healing mantra, attention may be placed on a part of the body that needs healing. Each mantra is repeated with a clear intention that amplifies its power and effect upon the body or mind. The combination of the energy inherent to the sound, the focus of attention and the focus of intention transforms a simple sound into a powerful tool for healing, as well as for the transformation of consciousness.

Below are a few classical mantras that invoke Divine blessings for peace and healing. The proper use of each mantra requires a teacher to assist you in how to properly pronounce the words. Often a student is initiated into the use of a mantra as the ceremony increases the energy of intention that flows through the words.

Om Namo Narayanaya: This mantra increases the qualities of the water element in one's consciousness. As the water element increases, so too do its nurturing, soothing and healing properties. As such, this mantra is repeated for the purpose of bringing peace, balance and healing to our own hearts and to the world around us. When repeated with attention on the heart and the clear intention to create peace, divine energy flows from above down and fills the heart with peace. The combination of the sound, attention on the heart and the intention to create peace not only affects the person who is repeating the mantra but all those who hear it. As the sound is chanted, its energy spreads out and enters the vibration of the environment. Even if the sound is not perceived with the ear, it can still be picked up by the consciousness of another person or group of people. Thus, when one person chants this mantra, their heart becomes more peaceful and so does their personal environment. When a community chants this mantra, each person's heart becomes more peaceful and the peacefulness of the community is raised. When many communities gather together to chant it, it supports peace within a country. When people all around the world from many countries chant this mantra, a vibration of peace permeates the planet. Thus, this mantra is the chant for world peace. It is the mantra of Sri Narayana, the deity and symbol of peace and balance.

Om Dhanvantara Murtaya Namaha: This mantra is repeated specifically for the purposes of activating healing energy and opening oneself up to knowledge about healing. When repeated with attention and intention, divine energy flows from above down and is utilized either for healing an illness or to enhance receptivity to knowledge about healing. Thus, it is a good mantra for students of healing arts to chant prior to study. When this mantra is chanted with attention placed at the heart, intuitive knowledge about healing is gained. When it is chanted with attention placed on the area of the ajna chakra (the point between the eyebrows), intellectual knowledge about healing is gained. When this mantra is chanted with attention on an area of the body in need of healing, prana or healing energy becomes focused at that point. This is the mantra of Sri Dhanvantari, the deity and symbol of healing.

Single-Syllable Elemental Mantras

There is a single-syllable mantra for each of the five elements that increases their properties within the body and mind. These are chanted with attention on different parts of the body. Each site is considered to be a storage site for the qualities of that element. These sites are at the locations of the first five chakras (a center of elemental energy that is the energetic equivalent of a nerve plexus). Each of the first five chakras corresponds to one element. Below are the elemental mantras. Spellings differ and so the two most common spellings are presented.

Lam (Lum): VP-K+

This is the earth element mantra, and the focal point is as the site of the first chakra, or muladhara chakra. It is located between the anus and the genitalia. In the ordinary person, chanting this mantra with focus and attention brings about greater grounding and decreases vata and pitta doshas. In the spiritually pure individual, chanting this mantra creates the ability to sustain spiritual awareness and present moment of consciousness.

Vam (Vum): VP-K+

This is the water element mantra, and the focal point is at the site of the second chakra, or svadhisthana chakra, located between the pubic bone and the navel. In the ordinary person, chanting this mantra with focus and attention brings about deeper feelings, desires and sensuality. This mantra is nourishing and decreases the vata and pitta doshas. In the spiritually pure individual, this mantra increases the desire to know and serve God and to be one with the Divine.

Ram (Rum): VK-P+

This is the fire element mantra, and the focal point is at the site of the third chakra, or manipura chakra, located between the navel and the sternum, at the solar plexus. In the ordinary person, chanting this mantra with focus and attention brings about greater personal focus and passion. This mantra decreases the vata and kapha doshas. In the spiritually pure individual, chanting this mantra brings about a greater capacity to fulfill one's divine dharma or spiritual purpose.

Yam (Yum): KP-V+

This is the air element mantra, and the focal point is at the site of the fourth chakra, or anahata chakra, located at the center of the breastbone or sternum. In the ordinary individual, chanting this mantra with focus and attention increases the movement of the mind and disperses energy throughout the body.

The mantra decreases the pitta and kapha doshas. In the spiritually pure individual, chanting this mantra cultivates detachment.

Ham (Hum): KP-V+

This is the ether element mantra, and the focal point is at the site of the fifth chakra, or vishudda chakra, located at the center of the throat. In the ordinary individual, chanting of this mantra with focus and attention increases self-expression. This is the expression of personal thoughts and ideas. This mantra pacifies the pitta and kapha doshas. In the person who is spiritually pure, chanting this mantra increases Self-expression or the expression of Divine understanding.

Om (Aum): PK-V+ (ex)

This is the mantra of realization, chanted with attention at the site of the sixth chakra, called ajna chakra, located at the central point between the eyebrows. It is also chanted with attention on the crown of the head, the location of the seventh chakra, or sahasra padma chakra. In the ordinary individual, chanting this mantra with attention and intention brings about greater mental clarity. It brings balance to pitta and kapha doshas and may be chanted by those with a vata nature as well as long as there is no serious imbalance in the dosha. In the spiritually pure individual, chanting this mantra harmonizes one's personal consciousness or awareness with the divine, thereby dissolving the barrier between the two. The sound itself is the unifying sound of the three primordial concepts of preservation (a), destruction (u), and creation (m). In the Hindu tradition, the sounds are symbols of Vishnu, Shiva and Brahma respectively. Chanting the sound returns awareness to an integrated state known as Brahman.

The Sound of Silence

As important as sound is for healing, silence, when used properly, is also a powerful tool. Silence increases the qualities of the ether element within the mind. The qualities of ether erase all disturbances in the mind. Ether empties the mind of thought, drama and imagination, returning it gradually to the inner silence of the present moment. When silence is achieved, the mind is clear and at peace and one's consciousness is filled with bliss.

It may not be possible for you to sustain complete silence. This is an ideal whose practice is reserved for great Masters. Most people's minds are filled with drama and that drama contributes to suffering. Even though complete silence may seem far away, taking periods of silence is very helpful. Each period of silence calms the mind down a little more creating greater clarity. Slowly, realizations emerge, as divine light begins to penetrate the disturbances. Each realization creates a shift in your consciousness and changes your experience of life.

Silence Exercise

Take one hour to be in complete silence. Go to a quiet place. It could be in your home if you feel at peace there or you may choose to go to a park. Go somewhere where you are not likely to be interrupted. During that hour, do not talk or write. This will begin the process of making the mind less active. Do not expose your mind to noises other than those of nature. Avoid all television, radio and music during this time. Do not read either, as this simply distracts your mind from your dramas by creating an alternative drama. If there is nothing to do, what will you do? You might choose to just sit quietly and experience your surroundings. You might chose to lay down on the grass and look up at the sky or close your eyes and allow the sun to bathe you. You may also choose to meditate. At first, your mind will wander about. As time passes and with repeated practice, it will slow down and greater stillness and its benefits will be known. Each time you do this, you will go deeper and deeper. With experience, increase the time you spend in silence.

Additional Methods for Creating Silence

- Find a place to watch the sun rise or set. Sit quietly and watch the show that is before your eyes. It is different every night.

- Take a 20 minute walk by yourself at lunch time to allow your mind to settle.

- Commit yourself to 24 hours without listening to the television, radio or any other entertainment device.

- Take method number three a step further and do not read during this time either. Reading will cause your mind to engage in the dramas of the world or of a fictional world.

- Commit yourself for 24 hours to not speak. Take this a step further and do not allow others to speak to you for the same 24 hours. You may need to go on a retreat or stay in your home for this to happen.

- Take up a meditation practice. There are many styles and almost all are beneficial for cultivating inner silence.

Personal Reflections

Sound has been a very important part of my life, particularly in the form of music. As a teenager and throughout my early adult years, I listened to a lot of music. I was attracted to rock and roll in my middle and late teens and that interest eventually morphed into a love of the Grateful Dead as well as a broad interest in jazz and world music. I found that music could transform my thoughts, feelings and emotions. It could make me feel good. The mystical side of the Grateful Dead intrigued me. When I closed my eyes, their music could carry me into altered states of consciousness. While the music was associated with the use of psychedelic drugs, with or without the drugs, the music clearly changed the biochemistry of my brain, opening my mind to new ideas and new ways of experiencing myself and my relationship to the world around me. Listening to the Grateful Dead was for me an early form of meditation. For those who are interested, the transcendental music of the Grateful Dead is rich in the elements ether and air. In general, it is expansive, mobile and flowing and is neither cooling nor warming. The music is generally more beneficial to pitta and kapha doshas but is not grounding enough to bring balance to vata dosha.

LESSON 13: HEALING YOUR LIFE THROUGH TOUCH

With your hands, touch my body. With your words, touch my mind. With your love, touch my soul.

We are just as affected by how we are touched as we are by what we eat, smell, see and hear. A touch can be healing or a touch can cause harm. If what we take in through our sense of touch is harmonious, our body and mind develop the physiology of health. If what we take in is disharmonious, our body and mind move toward disease. The art of ayurvedic touch therapy is the art of knowing what type of touch will bring harmony and healing to you and then bringing this type of touch into your life.

It may be difficult to think of touch as essential to your well-being. However, just as you could starve if you received no food, you could also starve if you received no touch. Studies show that babies who are not touched have a lower chance of survival and are often delayed in their development. Dr. Tiffany Field from the University of Miami School of Medicine, a leading researcher in the field of the effects of touch, states that touch is the first sense to develop and the last to fade even after sight, hearing, smell and taste have faded with age. Her work and that of her colleagues has been published in major medical journals including: Early Childhood Development and Care; Research in Nursing and Health; and Child Development. The following is just a partial list of the benefits of touch that have been published:

- Touch reduces aggressive tendencies
- Touch stimulates growth and development in children
- Touch helps children who are upset to calm down
- Massage of autistic children decreases their disruptive behaviors
- Massage improves relaxation leading to improved sleep
- Massage improves alertness
- Massage reduces pain in the body
- Massage improves immune function and specifically increases T-cells that fight cancer and viruses
- Massage increases the levels of dopamine and serotonin, two brain chemicals that improve mental outlook.
- Touch reduces cortisol levels in the body. Cortisol is a hormone that rises when we are under stress. Thus, touch appears to reduce stress.

It is widely accepted that touch plays an important role in the physical and psychological development of a new-born child. Touch has been found to stimulate the nervous system, the immune system, the muscular system, the circulatory system and brain development. A child who is not appropriately touched often enough is not likely to develop in a healthy manner. According to renowned child development expert, Dr. William Sears, "We believe every baby has a critical level of need for touch and nurturing in order to thrive." Dr. Sears goes on to describe thriving as not just getting bigger, but growing to one's potential, physically and emotionally.

In 1994, a study was published in the Journal of the American Academy of Child and Adolescent Psychiatry (1994 Oct; 33(8): 1098-105). This study revealed that mothers of children with a failure to thrive provide less matter-of-fact touch while feeding and also less unintentional touch during play. This suggests that mothers may unintentionally contribute to their child's failure to thrive due do an aversion to touch on the part of either the mother or the child.

The Broad Spectrum of Touch

While it is clear that touch has positive health benefits, it would be unwise to conclude that all touch has the same positive effects. Ayurveda emphasizes that we each have unique reactions to sensory stimulation based upon our constitution and the nature of any imbalances that are present. Just as different foods have different effects upon the body, so too do different types of touch. Just as junk food can make us sick, so too can junk touch. Though we may survive on it, we do not thrive on it and over time, it can contribute to disease.

Along the broad spectrum of touch lies junk touch on one end and healing touch on the other. In between lie a multitude of touch types. An example of an extreme junk touch experience is one that causes immediate harm, such as being struck by a rock or a fist. This produces immediate suffering. Junk touch is not always so extreme and its effects are not always immediate. Other examples of junk touch include that which occurs with contact sports, piercing of body parts, cutting of the skin and being pushed or slapped. These types of touch are rarely healing and are most often physically or emotionally destructive. Surprisingly though, some benefit is gained even from this type of touch. For some people, pain is necessary to allow a wounded psyche to feel like it is alive.

The effects of touch are cumulative over time. Eating candy once won't cause much suffering. However, if it is eaten often, it contributes to heart disease. Likewise, being slapped once may not cause much suffering (still not very good for you), but being slapped often can lead to deep feelings of betrayal, confusion, fear or anger and damage the psyche and through the mind-body connection, contribute to physical disease. Even mild disharmonious forms of touch damage the body and mind over time.

On the other end of the spectrum are the intentional healing touch techniques that have become common in alternative medicine. Techniques such as massage, polarity and reiki are good examples. A skilled touch therapist can support the healing of any physical or emotional condition. Yet, touch therapy is not only practiced by therapists. Perhaps the first touch therapy any of us received is from our parents when they hold and hug us when we are hurt. The healing touch of a parent as they rub a child's bruise is more than psychological. Rubbing a bruise or a bump has been proven to reduce pain by stimulating the nerves in the surrounding tissues. These stimulated nerves help block the signals of pain from the injured tissue reducing the perception of pain. It is no wonder that when we hurt ourselves the first things we do is touch, hold or rub the injured area!

Massage therapy is not the only way to receive a healing touch. Much less recognized is the benefit of a hug. Hugs have both physiological and emotional benefits. Studies out of The University of North Carolina at Chapel Hill looked at the effects of hugging on the physiology of the body. The researchers found that hugging increases the levels of oxytocin in the body. The more touch, the higher the levels. Oxytocin is a hormone known to participate in creating positive social bonding between two people. They also found that it reduced cortisol levels. Cortisol is a hormone that rises when we are under stress. The generally accepted conclusion is that hugging reduces stress and that this may decrease the incidence of all stress-related diseases while supporting the healing process.

Do you really need research to verify what you already know deep inside your own heart? It doesn't take a genius to come to the conclusion that touching and hugging are healthy. It does take brilliant researchers, however, to prove it and detail how it works. You also don't have to wait till all of the facts are in. You can benefit from it right away. Hugging is Universal Health Care. You just have to learn to ask nicely for a hug.

The Ayurvedic Art of Touch and Massage

The ayurvedic art of touch therapy is the art of matching up the type of touch to the person. Some people thrive on lots of touch and some on just a little. Some thrive on strong, deep touch and others on a gentle touch. Nothing is right for everyone and everything is right for someone. By understanding the qualities inherent in a specific type of touch, a type of touch can be applied based upon the qualities that will bring healing and harmony to the individual.

The Qualities of Touch

Hot / Cold: Touch is heating when the hands move quickly and cause friction to the skin. This occurs more quickly with a dry massage than when oil is used. It is easy to notice a heating massage as it turns the skin red. Deep pressure massages are also more heating. Slow and light movements of the hands are cooler, and so is a hug. Hot touches increase the influence of the fire element in the body. Cool touches decrease the influence of the fire element. Warm touch is best for vata and kapha doshas. Cool touch is best for bringing balance to pitta dosha.

Mobile / Stable: A mobile massage is one in which the therapist's hands move quickly. It increases the influence of the air element in the body. A stable massage is one in which the therapist's hands move slowly. It decreases the influence of the air element. A fast massage is stimulating and brings balance to kapha dosha. A slow massage is calming and is best for pacifying vata dosha. In general, the pitta dosha also benefits from a slower massage.

Dry / Moist: Moist massages take place with oils. Oils increase the qualities of the water element in the body. Dry massages take place without oils or with powders and decrease the influence of the water element. Some oils are moister than others. Sesame, almond and olive oils are very lubricating. Safflower and mustard oils are drier. Moist oil massage is best for balancing vata dosha but can increase the pitta and kapha doshas.

Heavy / Light: A heavy touch is strong and often occurs through the application of deep pressure. It increases the qualities of the earth element within the body. A light touch has a gentle and superficial effect. It increases the influence of the ether element in the body. A heavy massage is better for vata dosha. A light massage is best for kapha dosha. For those with a pitta constitution a moderate touch is often best.

Hard / Soft: A soft touch is gentle. A hard touch is not. The vata dosha benefits from soft touches. The kapha dosha benefits from harder touches. Pitta dosha is in between.

Rough / Smooth: A smooth massage takes place when oils are used. A rough massage takes place when oils are not used. A rough massage benefits the kapha dosha. A smooth massage benefits vata dosha. Pitta dosha is in between.

Gross / Subtle: A gross (large) touch touches a significant amount of the body at one time. A good example is a full body hug. A subtle touch makes contact with limited amount of the body at one time. A good example is stroking the skin lightly with the fingertips. A subtle touch increases the influence of the ether element. A gross touch increases the influence of the earth element. A gross touch is best for vata and pitta doshas. A subtle touch is best for kapha dosha.

Sharp / Dull: A sharp touch occurs when a narrow part of the body is used to do a massage and a dull touch occurs when a broad part of the body is used. Deep finger pressure, as occurs in trigger point therapy is sharp. The open hand is dull. Sharp massage is best for bringing healing to kapha dosha. Dull massage is best for bringing healing to vata and pitta doshas.

Cloudy / Clear: It is difficult to categorize a type of touch as cloudy or clear. It is easier to see this quality in the effect that it has on the mind of the recipient. A cloudy touch leaves a person's mind fuzzy at the end. A clear touch leaves a person's mind clear. Odd as it may seem, it is beneficial for a person of vata or pitta dosha to feel a little cloudier at the end of a massage session. This gives the mind a rest and stops it from perseverating and calculating. It is beneficial for a person of kapha nature to feel clearer after a massage.

Dense / Flowing: A dense massage focuses on one area of the body. A flowing massage moves gracefully from one part of the body to the next. A dense massage is best for vata and pitta doshas. A flowing massage is best for kapha dosha.

Types of Touch

Deep Tissue Massage: Trigger Points Therapy, Cross Fiber Therapy and Rolfing (K-V+ P+ (ex))

Deep massage applies a strong force to the body. As a result, the air element in the body of the receiver is increased. The fire element also increases when that force is focused and becomes sharper. This is particularly true when a single finger or elbow is used to apply the pressure to a local spot. The skin in the region will become reddened.

This force is excellent for removing physical and emotional stagnation and sluggishness. It is best for kapha dosha. It increases vata dosha and so is not recommended for those who are anxious, highly sensitive to their environment, in considerable pain or who have a low tolerance for discomfort. Individuals with a pitta nature benefit from a moderate pressure during massage, especially when there is ama (toxins) in the body and they are feeling strong (strong ojas).

Effleurage: Gentle Massage (VP-K+)

Gentle massage is the application of a light and slow force to the body. The massage has a greater predominance of the ether element inherent within it. When it is applied with full hand contact in a slow but flowing manner, it is appropriate for vata dosha, as this type of motion has greater water within it. When it is applied very lightly using the fingertips, the subtle quality of ether is increased and this is best for kapha dosha. Both types are fine for pitta dosha, as the stroke has a cooling nature. Gentle whole hand massage supports the rebuilding of the body's strength and is ideal for those individuals who feel weak, recovering from illness or exhausted. Gentle fingertip massage is best for those who are in need of inspiration.

Petrissage: Kneading and Wringing (K-PV+ (ex))

Kneading and wringing are moderate-to deep-massage strokes that push, pull, lift and torque the muscle belly. These strokes are slightly warming and a little mobile but become more warming and mobile the deeper and faster they are performed respectively. When performed slowly at a moderate depth, they are not very aggravating to any of the doshas while providing the greatest benefit to kapha dosha. When they are performed faster and deeper, they become aggravating to vata and pitta doshas while bringing even greater balance to kapha dosha.

Friction Massage (K-VP+)

In friction massage, the hands move quickly over the body. This increases the influence of air and fire elements and the body becomes hot and agitated. Friction strokes alleviate stagnation and sluggishness and are best for reducing the kapha dosha and for purifying the body. Those with a vata or pitta nature should avoid a massage that emphasizes this type of stroke.

Tickling (K-V+P (n))

Tickling is an experience of intense stimulation to the nerves of the body that does not cause immediate damage and is not strong enough to produce pain. The tickle has the qualities of being light, thin, subtle, sharp and mobile. These qualities reflect those of the air element and increase its influence in the body. If a person has a disturbance in the air element (vata imbalance) in their body or mind, it is not likely that they will enjoy being tickled very much. Tickling can be beneficial for reducing excess kapha but strongly increases vata. For a person of pitta nature, tickling can go either way. If pitta is out of balance, tickling is likely to make the person angry. If a person of pitta nature is in balance, however, it can be enjoyed and won't cause pitta to increase.

Tapotement: Tapping and Percussion (KV-P+)

Tapping on the body or percussion is a popular massage technique in which the body is used like a drum and the hands are the drum sticks. Either the outer edge of the hands is used or the hands are cupped at the palm. In general, this technique is mobile, dry and warm. Tapping and percussion are generally beneficial for reducing excess kapha dosha. It is excellent for loosening up mucus in the lungs, bringing stimulation to the nervous system and reducing lethargy. Care should be used in applying this stroke to those with a vata imbalance as it increases vata dosha. When performed very fast or with greater energy, these strokes become heating and increase pitta dosha as well.

Choosing the Best Oil for Your Massage

Massage can be performed with oils, powders or with nothing at all. Ayurvedic massage with oils has become quite popular and is now available at most spas around the world. Ayurvedic massage with oil is often called "snehana", which also means "to love". Indeed, the application of oil to the skin of the body is considered a very deep form of nourishment and builds the health of the immune and nervous systems of the body. The daily application of oil to the body builds self-love and the nurturing qualities that it increases support the expression of love toward others.

An important consideration is what type of oil to apply to the body and how much to apply. Oil contains considerable water and earth elements. Oils are generally moist, heavy, smooth and dull. Depending on the oil though, it can be warming or cooling. Some oils are considered less oily than others and do not greatly increase the moist quality of the body. Some are also lighter than others and contain less of the earth element. Those which are drier and lighter are best for people with a kapha nature.

Massage Oils Summary Table

Below is a description of several commonly available oils, their qualities and their effects upon the doshas when applied through massage.

Oil	Warming or Cooling	Other Qualities	Doshic Effects
*Sesame	Warm	Heavy, moist, dull, smooth, flowing	V-P+K=
*Almond	Warm	Heavy, moist, dull, flowing	V-P+K=
Canola	Cool	Light, dry	PK-V+
Sunflower	Cool	Light, moist, dull, smooth	P-VK+
Coconut	Cool	Heavy, moist, dull, smooth	P-VK+
Olive	Cool	Heavy, moist, dull, smooth	PV-K+
Safflower	Warm	Lighter, drier	K-P+V=
Mustard	Warm	Lighter, drier	K-VP+

*Sesame oil is generally considered the premier oil in Ayurveda. Although it has qualities that increase kapha dosha, it can still be used to treat kapha dosha, as it also has a strong flowing action that reduces the dense quality of kapha dosha. The same flowing quality is found in almond oil.

Massage and the Three Doshas
Touch and Massage for Vata

People with a vata nature or imbalance benefit from the soothing, calming, loving and nourishing aspects of touch. There is a need for nurturance. Hugs are very healing and so too is an oil massage that is calming, soothing and grounding.

The best strokes to receive during a massage are those that are slow (stable) with a light to moderate depth using a broad hand contact (gross, dull). This type of effleurage, along with light-to-moderate kneading, is very healing. Deep tissue massage is not supportive and should be avoided, as it is not nurturing and it creates too much pain. Those with a vata nature or imbalance are the most pain sensitive. Deep pressure points and elbow massage should certainly be avoided. Other types of touch that should be minimized or avoided all together include tapping, percussion, friction massage and tickling.

The best oil to use is refined sesame oil, as it is the most nourishing of all the oils. The next best is almond oil. By adding essential oils into the base oil, the oil can be made so that it has a pleasant aromatic quality as well.

Touch and Massage for Pitta

People with a pitta nature or imbalance also benefit from the nurturing quality of touch and massage. When a person with a pitta nature is burned out, more nurturance is needed to restore their energy. A hug helps to provide that nurturance and so does receiving a good massage.

The best strokes are those that are applied slowly with a broad hand contact. This type of effleurage is cooling and stable. It should be applied at a light or moderate depth but not too deep. The deeper the strokes are applied, the more heating they become. Pressure point and elbow massage should be minimized as they are too sharp and intense. Tapping and percussion are unnecessary to balance the dosha but kneading and wringing can be very beneficial. These should be performed slowly at a moderate depth.

It is interesting to note that people with a pitta nature often want deep massage. There is an acceptance of the "no pain, no gain" concept. This is because they are used to working hard and staying focused in order to get results. There is a belief that whatever will help should be done–even if it hurts. This attitude is more often part of what caused the problem and is less often the solution.

Coconut oil is a great oil to use during a massage. It is very nourishing (heavy) and is the best oil to use where there is weakness from burnout. Olive and sunflower, though cooling, are a little lighter and better for maintenance and long-term use. Cooling essential oils may be added to the mix to make the oil more pleasing.

If a person of pitta nature has lots of ama (toxin) within, then more purification is needed. You can tell if more purification is necessary by looking at the tongue. If your tongue has a moderate or thick yellow coating, then purification is best so long as you are not too weak from burnout. When purification is needed, sunflower oil is the best oil to use as it is lighter. In addition, deeper strokes can be applied though they should be applied very slowly. Deeper strokes loosen up the toxins allowing them to circulate and be eliminated by the body.

Touch and Massage for Kapha

People with a kapha nature or imbalance benefit from more purification through touch and massage. While loving hugs are always appreciated, they will not have the same healing effect on people with kapha imbalances. For healing purposes, a strong, deep touch is needed and the hands should move quickly over the body.

The best strokes to receive are deep tissue, petrissage and friction massage. These strokes are stimulating and purifying helping to remove stagnation and toxic buildup. As those with a kapha nature generally have the highest pain tolerance, deep tissue massage is better received. Tapping and percussion are also quite healing, as well as providing stimulation while loosening up mucus and additional toxins.

The best oils to use are a mixture of safflower and mustard as they are the lightest and driest of the oils. Stimulating essential oils may be added to make the oil more pleasing and potent. However, no oil is necessary and a dry powder massage is quite beneficial. While any powder can be used, a powder prepared from chickpeas mixed with a blend of calamus, clove and bayberry is ideal.

Methods to Bring the Healing Touch into Your Life
Go Get a Massage
Massage therapy is available in almost every part of the world today. There are many styles of massage therapy and different forms are best for different types of people and different conditions. Select a massage therapist who can bring the proper form of healing touch to you. Because receiving a massage is often a multi-sensory experience, ask that the music played in the room and the type of aroma therapy provided be in alignment with your needs.

Self Oil Massage (Self-Abhyanga)
While receiving a massage is a beautiful and healing experience, giving yourself a massage is even more healing. Perhaps this is because it is free and you can give yourself one every day. This allows the healing benefits of the oils and the massage to build up over a long period of time. In Ayurveda, a daily self oil massage is considered essential to creating optimal health.

Self oil massage is immediately beneficial to your skin, your muscles and your nervous system. Over time, all of the tissues of your body benefit. As important as these benefits are, the most important benefit comes from showing love for yourself. If your ojas (energy reserve) is low, you will find yourself depleted, irritable, easily angered, anxious, nervous or overly controlling. In this state, your capacity to show love (kindness, compassion) and nurture others is diminished. When you place oil on your body, you are feeding yourself and restoring your capacity to love yourself (be kind and compassionate) and to share that love with others.

Below are instructions for a daily self oil massage practice.

Ayurvedic Method of Self Oil Massage
- Purchase high quality oil (cold-processed, organic) from a health food store that balances the dosha that is most out of balance.
- Purchase an 8 oz. bottle (glass is best)
- Pour the oil into the bottle. Store the rest of the oil in a cool, dark place for maximum shelf life.
- If you wish, add appropriate essential oils (see aromatherapy

section) to the bottle.

- Warm up the oil before each application. You can either place the bottle inside a sauce pan that has been filled with hot water or place the bottle in a sink full of hot water that has been plugged to prevent the water from going down the drain.

- Warm the oil until it is comfortably warm but not too hot. Put a little on your wrist to test it.

- Apply the oil to your body: Pour some in your hands. Use it liberally. Use both hands to spread it along the body part. Use long strokes to cover an entire leg or arm. Use circular strokes around the joints of the body. You will notice that the warm oil spreads easily. Keep rubbing it in. Let your body soak it up. The absorption of oil is very important in order to restore balance. If you are of kapha nature, use faster and deeper strokes as you apply it. If you are of vata or pitta nature, start with some quick strokes to help the oil absorb but then go slowly and gently.

- If possible, let the rest of the oil absorb into your body for the next 20 minutes or more. This is a good time for meditation or yoga practice.

- If needed: Take a towel and pat off the excess oil. Try not to wash it off with soap as that will deplete the skin of oil.

- If there is not enough time to let the oil completely absorb, either use less oil so that you do not stain your clothing when you put it on or use an oil such as almond oil that absorbs more quickly.

- If you shower after the massage, try to wait at least 20 minutes to allow for maximum absorption.

- If you place oil on your body after a shower, that is fine too but if you do not allow it to absorb, it could stain your clothes. This can be avoided with a lighter coating of oil.

For a person with a vata or pitta nature, this practice helps to restore strength and build resistance to disease. For those with a kapha nature, this practice helps to awaken the body and mind while stimulating the nervous and circulatory systems.

LESSON 14: THE HEALING RHYTHMS OF DAILY LIFE

In the celestial dance, the sun and moon are our partners.

Our daily routines are the foundation upon which our health rests. Less glamorous than the sensory therapies, it is often ignored. Its beauty lies hidden beneath the rigid exterior of discipline. As its exterior softens, a rhythm emerges and harmony flows effortlessly in step with the cosmic dance. In that moment, its beauty shines through you for all to see.

I may be addressing it last but it comes first in overall importance to well-being. Your daily routines reflect the sum total of how you live your life. If you have healthy routines, you will have a healthy life, your inner beauty will shine and you will reach more of your full potential. If you have unhealthy routines, your foundation will eventually crack, your health and well-being will suffer and that light that illuminates your inner beauty will fade. No matter how beautiful your body, when that light fades, only a hard shell of your former self remains. How do you live each day? What time do you wake up and go to bed and what happens in-between? What is the rhythm of your day? With whom do you dance?

Health is a rhythm. If you dance or play music, you know the feeling of being in rhythm with other musicians and the odd feeling of being out of sync. When you are in sync, the music takes on a life of its own. It enters inside of you and moves your body. The music dances the dancer. It plays the musician. When you are out of rhythm, there is a sense of struggle as you try to find your way back. Health is very similar. The difference is that with health you need to be in rhythm with all of nature, especially the sun and moon. When we are in rhythm, we flow effortlessly through life. When we are out of rhythm, we stumble into ill health and our well-being suffers. It takes effort to bring us back into harmony.

There are some general factors that affect everyone, such as the rhythms of night and day. However, each person also has their own unique internal rhythms. This is why there is no one rhythm that is ideal for everyone. We are all unique. The discovery of your own unique internal rhythms and how to restore your connection to the rhythm of nature can be made through an understanding of your constitution. Without this knowledge, you are likely to fall into a rhythm that is dictated by society, the people around you or the desires of your ego.

The Healing Rhythm of Vata

The tendency of a person with a vata constitution is to be erratic. Change and inconsistency is common. As a result, regular routines are important but difficult to create. Vata dosha, consisting of air and ether, does not have a natural container. Vata moves like the wind and changes direction often. Being light and subtle, less attached and less focused, people with a vata nature are easily affected by the influences surrounding them and, as such, are most likely to adapt to the rhythms (healthy or unhealthy) of the people around them. While this trait makes them easy to get along with, it also has some unfortunate side effects.

When a person with a vata nature lacks a consistent rhythm, the mobile nature of vata dosha increases. This disturbs the body's internal energy, called prana, leading to greater internal anxiety, nervousness, confusion, feelings of overwhelm and restlessness and an inability to follow through on plans and projects. In addition, as the internal movement of prana increases, the body and mind become drier. This is similar to what happens to the skin when you stand in the wind. Ayurveda teaches that the fluid of the body, called rasa, is essential not only for hydrating the tissues of our body but also for nourishing our mind. Dryness leads to greater dissatisfaction in life, irritability, hardness and rigidity. The combination of excessive motion and dryness leads to an increase in the light quality. This causes the body and mind to become depleted over time and there is a loss of the ability to endure stress (low ojas).

Vata requires a container to hold its energy. Stable, regular routines help to channel and focus the great amount of natural energy (prana) that a person with a vata nature has. When stable routines are present, not only does the body perform better but the mind is calmer. Sleep is easier and performance in life is more effective. Within the structure of stable routines, a person of vata nature is able to accomplish a great deal within a very short period of time. In fact, when structure is present, a person of vata nature can be more productive than any other individual doshic type.

The healing rhythm for a person with a vata nature or imbalance is a steady rhythm with few fluctuations. Regular routines are essential to their well-being. Regular rhythms surrounding sleeping, eating and working each day creates the structure that energy (prana) can flow through.

The Healing Rhythm of Pitta

The nature of pitta is to be focused. Pitta, consisting mostly of fire, is sharp and can be intense. Contained within water, a person with a pitta tendency is able to sustain their focus. When they move forward, they do so with conviction. While this trait makes them natural leaders, it also has some unfortunate side effects.

The focused and intense nature of a person with a pitta constitution increases pitta's natural sharp and hot qualities. Eventually, if the pitta dosha is not pacified, a person will tend to burn out. Ayurveda teaches that the red blood cells of the body are the source of invigoration. Red blood cells carry fiery hemoglobin, which transports oxygen to the tissues of the body, providing them with energy. When pitta rises, the body becomes very efficient, not only in its use of oxygen but in its use of all metabolic substances, resulting in a lean, mean machine. At first, there is a sense of power and strength, but when it is on-going, the body overheats and fatigues, like an engine that starts steaming after working too hard. In the body, the excess heat causes a host of challenges as it spreads into the tissues, most notably inflammation.

People with a pitta nature are planners. Planning emerges as natural outgrowth of a focused nature and leads to achievement. A person with a pitta nature likes to know the routine and to follow the routine as long as they believe that the routine will lead them to the goal. While focused on the goal, they are not overly attached to the routine and will change it whenever new information comes along that leads them to believe that there is a better way. The mind of a person with a pitta nature is always calculating the odds of success and making adjustments.

Regular routines are healthy for a person with pitta nature. It strengthens the foundation under their feet allowing for greater success without greater stress. Routines increase the quality of the water and earth elements allowing for sustainability. Regular routines protect a person of pitta nature from the intensity of their own fire.

The healing rhythm of a person with a pitta nature or imbalance is a steady rhythm that allows for flexibility and fluctuations. While regular routines are essential to their well-being, occasional spontaneity is also very healthy. While sleeping, eating, working and playing at the same or similar times each day creates a supportive structure that protects against the heat and intensity of the fire, a spontaneous adventure once in a while is important and helps to break the intensity.

The Healing Rhythm of Kapha

The nature of kapha is to be steady and move slowly. Consisting of water and earth, kapha dosha has the qualities of mud. It is soft, heavy and slow, and provides for a solid structure supporting regular steady routines. In fact, the routines of a person with a kapha nature can become so steady they form a rut that is hard to get out of. This is because, as water and earth combine together, they form a sticky quality. We could call the sticky quality, "attachment." It binds a person to one way of doing things. The routine is preferred, not because it is necessarily the best, but because it has always been followed in the past. This sticky quality makes it difficult for a person with a kapha nature to be spontaneous or to change their routine.

This sticky or attached quality has benefits and challenges for a person with a kapha nature. On the one hand, it leads to reliability and dependability. On the other hand, a lifestyle based on repetitive routines continues to increase the water and earth elements. This leads to a continuing increase in the qualities of kapha. Over time, the body and mind become more and more stagnant.

Physically, there is an increase in weight and mucus formation. Psychologically, there is a loss of motivation, inspiration and decrease in general excitement.

In order to stay in balance, a person with a kapha nature needs to break the steadiness of their daily rhythm. While a daily rhythm supports well-being in general, a person with a kapha nature benefits from greater spontaneity. Spontaneity increases the air element in the body and supports both dryness and mobility, two qualities that help to keep kapha dosha in balance.

The Rhythm of Sleep and Rest

Sleep and rest is heavy, moist and stable. It rejuvenates the body and helps restore a positive outlook on life.

A healthy sleep rhythm is based on an alignment between our body and the movements of the sun. As the sun rises, our natural bodily energy should begin to be aroused. As the sun sets, our natural bodily energy should begin to calm down and prepare for sleep. This rhythm is based on our connection with light. Light is warming and mobile, it illuminates and awakens the body and mind. Darkness is cooling and stable, it sedates the mind helping to prepare for sleep.

When you are living in rhythm with light and darkness, you will tend to awaken early and become tired earlier in the evening. Many people experience this when they go camping and get away from the artificial rhythms of light they are usually exposed to. Living with this natural rhythm is very healthy. Ayurveda considers proper sleep and rest to be one of the pillars of life (proper rest, proper digestion and proper use of sexual energy). If we are sleeping and resting well, we will experience greater health. When we are not, our well-being suffers.

Healthy Sleep and Waking Rhythm for Vata Dosha

If you have a vata imbalance, you may be having difficulty falling to sleep. This is one of the most common signs of a vata imbalance. Often, it is difficult to slow the mind down enough to sleep. There may be worry or anxiety or there may simply be too much creative energy surging through the mind. In addition, the body may be restless. You may feel like tossing and turning, you may feel that energy is building up in your legs, arms or stomach. This condition is called Restless Leg Syndrome.

A proper sleeping and waking routine is important to keep vata dosha in balance and to prevent further symptoms of vata disturbance. For starters, it is important to go to bed and wake up at or about the same time every day. Depending upon the time of year and where in the world you live, the sun will set at different times. As a general rule, going to sleep at about 10:00 pm is appropriate. If you live in an area with more light, this time can be pushed forward one hour. If you live in an area with very little light, this time can be moved backward one hour. Thus, in the wintertime, it is best to go to bed a little earlier and in the summertime, a little later. In order to be able to fall asleep at the appropriate time, it is necessary to have awoken at the proper time. Otherwise, you might not be tired. The proper time to wake up is at sunrise. Yes, sunrise! Even if you had a difficult time sleeping, it is still important to get up at sunrise so that your internal rhythms are not thrown too far off. If you do, it is much more likely that you will fall asleep and sleep well the next night. The only time where sleeping in late or in the afternoon is healthy is when your body is greatly fatigued by severe stress or illness.

Proper rest is important to help keep a person with a vata nature in balance. Rest is rejuvenating and has a heavy, stable quality that preserves internal moisture. This balances vata's mobile, dry and light tendencies.

Having a Challenge Sleeping?
Try these practices to help restore your natural sleep rhythm

- Awaken at the appropriate time each morning even if you did not sleep well the night before.

- Sleep with the shades open to allow natural light to help awaken you in the morning.

- In the evening, avoid artificial light and use candlelight after the sun has gone down.

- If you are noise sensitive, practice using earplugs.

- Avoid working at night past 7:00 pm. Allow the mind a chance to rest before bed.

- Avoid computers after 7:00 pm as they agitate the energy of the body and mind.

- Watch only light comedies in the evening on television and turn it off by 8:00 pm.

- Consider a ½ hour of gentle yoga postures about 1 hour before bed.

- Make sure that you follow the other proper daily routines as they help avoid agitating your internal energy.

- Consider a glass of hot milk one hour before bed with 1/8 teaspoon of nutmeg or the ayurvedic herbs ashwagandha and jatamansi.

Healthy Sleep and Waking Rhythm for Pitta Dosha

If you have a pitta nature, most of the time you sleep well and awaken eager to engage the day's activities. However, when the stress level rises, you may find yourself unable to sleep as your mind works overtime planning for a solution to the problem at hand. Warm nights make it difficult to sleep as well.

A healthy sleep routine for a person with a pitta nature means going to bed at or around 10:00 pm and awakening ½ hour before the sun rises. Yes, before the sun rises, as the first rays of the morning light crack the dawn and the skies become lighter. As noted previously, if you live in an area with longer daylight, you should go to bed a little later. If you live in an area with shorter days, go to bed a little earlier. The same holds true for the shorter days of winter and the longer days of summer.

Rest is important to help keep a person with a pitta nature in balance and to prevent burnout. The heavy, cooling and stable qualities of rest temper pitta's fiery heat. If a person with a pitta nature is burned out, an afternoon nap can be beneficial. However, a person of pitta nature who is healthy should avoid afternoon naps as this works against the natural rhythm of nature.

Healthy Sleep and Waking Routines for Kapha Dosha

If you have a kapha nature or imbalance, chances are that sleep is not too difficult for you. Shortly after putting your head on the pillow, you are fast asleep. In fact, as kapha becomes more and more out of balance, sleep becomes easier and deeper and it can become difficult to wake up.

As sleep increases the heavy and stable qualities, too much sleep increases kapha dosha and contributes to imbalances. As a result, individuals with a kapha nature or imbalance benefit from less sleep and less rest than others. While the ideal time to go to bed is around 10:00pm, the ideal time to wake up is one hour before the sun rises. Awakening early and starting the day increases the mobile quality (air) and the warming quality (fire). This increases motivation and focus throughout the day. As noted previously, if you live in an area with longer daylight, you should go to bed a little later. If you live in an area with shorter days, go to bed a little earlier. The same holds true for the shorter days of winter and the longer days of summer.

The Healthy Morning Rhythm

For many people, the rhythm of the morning routine is the most challenging of all. Most people awaken with just enough time to accomplish the minimum amount of preparation for the day. For some, it is a quick shower and brushing of the teeth, then getting dressed and jumping into the car for breakfast on the go and a long commute to work. This is compounded if there are kids at home and we add in making breakfast for them, packing a lunch box and getting them out the door and to where they need to be. This type of hectic morning is not healthy. Rushing in the morning concerned about getting out on time produces stress and tension, weakening the body and disturbing the mind.

A healthy morning rhythm sets the stage for a peaceful, balanced and even more productive day. In order to establish this routine, however, it is essential to awaken early. And to awaken early, it is essential to go to bed early.

Imagine a morning routine that left time for calmly making breakfast and sitting down to eat it. Now imagine that it was possible to have time in the morning for meditation or reflection, yoga or tai-chi. How do you think the rest of your day would go? I can tell you how. You would be calmer and more relaxed. Your interactions with people would be more positive and you would be more focused and productive. In addition, you would have more energy to accomplish your goals and you would get sick less often. You would get all of these benefits for the small price of going to bed earlier and getting up earlier!

An ayurvedic morning routine begins with waking up early and then incorporates practices that support well-being. In addition to yoga and meditation, morning practices include self oil massage, nasal cleaning, proper evacuation of the bowels, and eye and tongue cleaning, along with the more typical routines of proper hygiene, such as brushing and flossing the teeth and taking a shower. Let's take a look at some of these practices.

The Morning Bowel Movement

A bowel movement every morning is important for general health and well-being. A morning bowel movement helps the body feel lighter and eliminates toxins from the body. If you eliminate regularly in the morning, you will be healthier and have a greater positive mental attitude. A morning bowel movement also allows you to deepen your practice of yoga and meditation.

Regardless of your constitution, a morning bowel movement is healthy. It is common for those with a vata imbalance to have the greatest difficulty with this, as vata dosha causes the bowels to become dry, hard and irregular or constipated. It is common for those with a vata imbalance to skip one or two days. However, this is an imbalance that can be corrected through proper eating habits and proper food choices, as previously described and by a regular and steady morning and daily rhythm.

One practice to help assure a morning bowel movement is to slowly drink an 8 ounce glass of warm water after you wake up. Then, go to the bathroom and sit on the toilet, whether you feel the urge to go or not. If your body is not used to evacuating your bowels in the morning, at first, nothing may happen. Sit quietly anyway for five minutes. This helps encourage the downward flow of energy called apana vayu. Be careful not to strain. Allow the urge to arise naturally. If you do not go, get up and get on with your morning activities. Repeat this daily along with the other routines and eventually the natural rhythm will restore itself.

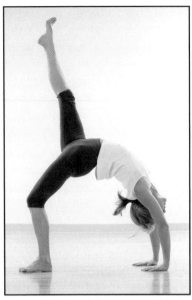

Yoga

It is beyond the scope of this book to explain the practices of yoga in any detail. The ayurvedic approach to yoga, however, alters the practices of yoga postures to meet the individual needs of each person in accordance with their constitution and the nature of any imbalances that might be present. If you are already practicing yoga postures, a few modifications to your practice may significantly improve your well-being. If you are not already practicing yoga, consider taking some yoga classes to learn. Once you learn how to perform the postures, practice every morning for at least 30 minutes. Yoga is best for you when you practice daily.

Those of you with a vata nature or imbalance should practice in a slow and calming manner, with attention on your connection to the earth. This will help to keep you grounded and to prevent excess mobility in your mind. Those with a pitta nature or imbalance should also practice slowly and with calm. You should not overheat yourself while practicing. This will help to keep you less intense and more relaxed. Those with a kapha nature or imbalance benefit from a practice that incorporates more movement from one posture to the next with shorter periods of relaxation between poses. This type of practice is more heating and mobile and helps to keep you in greater balance.

If you do not have a yoga practice, look for a local yoga studio and take a few different yoga classes until you find the class and the teacher that feels right to you. Every class and teacher is different. If you do not have a positive experience with your first class, don't give up. Most teachers will let you sample their classes for free. Keep sampling till you feel the right connection. Remember that classes are for the purpose of learning. Once you learn, take your practice away from the studio and incorporate it into your daily routine. Go back to classes from time to time to deepen your practice.

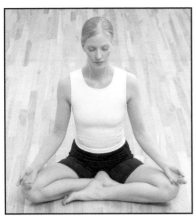

Meditation

Meditation is the practice of consciously focusing and calming the mind. There are many styles of meditation. Some include focusing inward on your breath or a mantra while others suggest witnessing the stream of thoughts that flow through the mind as if you were an observer sitting on the bank of a river watching the waters flow. The method that you use is less important than the regularity of your practice. A regular practice keeps the mind steady and calm and has been proven through scientific research to improve both physical and mental health.

If you do not already have a meditation practice, I suggest taking a local meditation class. Classes are offered in many communities and often your local yoga center can inform you of where you can take classes. Once again, learn in class and then take your meditation practice away from the classroom and incorporate it into your daily morning practice. Your morning meditation practice should last at least 15 minutes. However, start out slowly. If you find a longer practice difficult, begin with just 2-3 minutes of meditation in the morning. Your practice will naturally grow. Just be consistent. If you are doing well and your time in the morning allows you to meditate for a longer period of time, increase your practice to 30 minutes.

*Please note that meditation is contra-indicated for individuals with severe and borderline severe psychological disorders or tendencies toward such disorders without the guidance of a properly trained teacher of Ayurveda and yoga. These conditions include but are not limited to schizophrenia, bi-polar disorder, psychosis and depression.

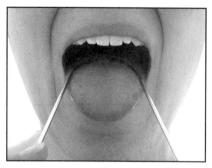

Tongue Cleaning

With the growth in awareness of Ayurveda, cleaning the tongue has entered the mainstream. Dentists now recommend it and tongue cleaners are available at many local drugstores. Cleaning the tongue in the morning improves the breath and Ayurveda teaches that via reflexes from the tongue, it also massages the organs helping to eliminate toxins from the body. The practice only takes 10-15 seconds and is usually performed at the same time as brushing the teeth. Using an actual tongue scrapper (often made from silver, stainless steel or copper) is more effective than using a toothbrush. Tongue cleaning is easy to perform, just move the instrument from the back of the tongue to the front 5-10 times. It is not necessary to use great pressure on the tongue and the practice should be very comfortable.

When you clean the tongue, it is likely that you will remove a thin coating on the tongue. The coating is often white and may be tinted yellow, green or gray. This is called ama in Ayurveda and is indicative of poor digestion and the buildup of toxins. As your digestion improves from following the proper diet and lifestyle, you will not produce a coating.

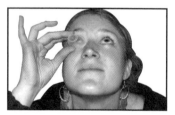

Eye Cleansing

The eyes are given a bath one at a time using an eye cup filled with a warm herbal solution. There are several herbal solutions that can be used. One of the easiest to use is rose water. Rose hydrosol (prepared from the water left over from the process of distilling rose essential oil) is available in most health food stores. If you keep an 8 ounce bottle by your sink, the process will not take very long. Just follow these directions.

- Fill the eye cup (available at your local drugstore) half way with the rose water.

- Fill the rest of the cup with warm water (tap or purified) so that the solution is near to body temperature. Look down into the cup as you place it to your eye.
- Keeping the seal to your skin, lift your head up and raise the cup toward the ceiling.
- Blink your eye slowly several times.
- Look down and remove the cup.
- Repeat on your other eye.

The practice only takes about a minute. It keeps the eye cool, removes morning mucus and is understood in Ayurveda to protect the vision when practiced regularly. It also helps to reduce itching and redness that accompanies allergies and minor infections.

Stronger solutions are sometimes prepared from an infusion of chrysanthemum flowers or the ayurvedic herbal formulation called triphala. Triphala is a mixture of dried powders of three fruits grown in India called amalaki, bibhitaki and haritaki.

If you experience allergies that affect your eyes or if you have mucus in your eyes in the morning, perform this practice daily or more often as needed. If you do not have these symptoms, this practice only needs to be performed once per week for the prevention of eye disease.

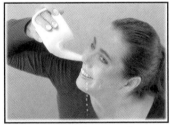

Nasal Cleansing

Cleansing the nasal passages is performed using a neti pot. Proper cleansing of the nostrils reduces the accumulation of airborne toxins and pollens. It improves the ability to breathe through the nose and reduces allergic symptoms. Following the cleansing, it is important to place a drop of oil (sesame) on the fingertip and apply it as deep as you can to the inside of the nostril. Keeping the nostril clean and slightly oily is considered important for improving the ability to absorb prana (life energy) from the breath. The oil also prevents dryness and protects the respiratory system from infection. When the nasal passages are working optimally, you will feel a higher level of invigoration throughout the day and have a more positive nature overall.

A neti pot is a small special tea pot with a spout that fits into the nostril. Neti pots are available in some drugstores, most health food stores, through any ayurvedic practitioner and online. Once you get your pot, follow these basic directions.

- Fill the pot with warm water at about body temperature (98-100 degrees).
- Add salt to the water. The amount varies with the size of the pot. In general, start with ½ tsp.
- Lean over the sink.
- Place the spout inside one nostril.
- Open and breathe through your mouth to equalize pressure. This is very important.
- Tip the pot into your nostril as you tilt your head forward and then turn to the side.
- Adjust yourself to allow the water to flow effortlessly from the pot into your nostril, around the nasal septum and out the opposite nostril. Use one pot full.
- Gently blow your nose.
- Repeat on the opposite side.
- Place one drop of sesame oil on your finger and apply it to the inside of the nostril.

This is an easier practice than it might seem. Once you learn how to do this, it does not take much effort and it is quite comfortable. If you experience discomfort, consider the following:

- Adjust the water temperature. If it is too hot, it will burn. If it is too cold, it will sting and may give you a headache as the water enters your sinuses.
- Adjust the salt concentration: Too much or too little will also sting and can give you a headache.
- Always remember to keep your mouth open as you perform this practice.

Self Oil Massage (Abhyanga)

This practice was described in detail in Lesson 13: Healing Your Life Through Touch. Self oil massage is very important for building the strength of the body and protecting the skin against dryness and heat. Over time, it helps to keep the skin healthy and looking young. The practice takes about ten minutes in the morning and is best performed before yoga and meditation and before a shower to allow as much oil as possible to be absorbed into the body. However, it can be lightly applied after a shower as well.

Always apply the oil once it has been warmed up. Oil massage is essential to the well-being of those with a vata nature or imbalance. It also benefits pitta dosha. Those with a kapha dosha or imbalance can use a lighter oil application or perform a dry massage for stimulation. See Lesson 13: Healing Your Life Through Touch for the specific types of oil to use to bring balance to each dosha.

Meals and Snacks

The proper rhythm for meals and snack times vary according to the constitution and nature of any imbalances that are present. If the proper rhythm for your constitution is not followed, you are very likely to develop symptoms of imbalance.

Vata's Rhythm for Meals and Snacks

It is healthiest for a person with a vata nature or imbalance to eat meals at regular, consistent times each day. This may be challenging for vata's mobile, irregular tendencies but it is essential to well-being.

People with a vata nature or imbalance benefit from eating five smaller meals each day. That is not a misprint. Five meals each day! Of course, we must remember to follow the rules for proper consumption. Each meal should be modest and leave you feeling 75% full. The meals are small in general, as the digestion of a person with a vata imbalance is often not very strong.

In order to eat five meals per day, a person of vata tendency should eat every three hours such as at 7, 10, 1, 4 and 7 o'clock. If you like a slightly more substantial breakfast, lunch and dinner, then the 10:00 and 4:00 meals can be lighter, healthy snacks. If these times do not work well for your schedule, you can modify them a little. But remember, you need to eat at or around the same time every day. A regular, consistent schedule of taking food will also prevent blood sugar abnormalities (high and low blood sugar levels) that are the cause of many emotional fluctuations, especially anxiety.

Pitta's Rhythm for Meals and Snacks

It is healthiest for a person with a pitta nature or imbalance to eat three substantial meals per day and avoid snacking between meals. Each meal should be larger than those that a person of vata or kapha nature might take. This is because the strength of digestion of a person with a pitta nature is stronger. Still, the meal should only leave you feeling 75% full.

Each meal should be spaced apart by about five hours. Meal times of 7:00 - 12:00 and 5:00 are very reasonable. While you can create your own schedule, try not to space your meals out too far or your hunger level will rise and you will find yourself becoming more critical and irritable. In addition, be sure to avoid eating within three hours of going to bed to allow food to digest properly. Remember, be consistent.

Kapha's Rhythm for Meals and Snacks

An individual with a kapha nature or imbalance, having slower digestion and a tendency toward becoming heavy, benefits from eating less frequently and consuming a smaller quantity of food. It is healthiest to eat only two meals per day about eight hours apart.

The first meal, which should be the larger of the two, is best taken at around 10:00 am. This is the time that the sun is beginning to march toward its peak. At this time, the strength of the digestive fire naturally rises, making it easier to digest food. The second meal, a little lighter, should be taken at 6:00 pm. This will have allowed plenty of time for the previous meal to have digested properly. Pay attention to how you feel when you eat and make sure that when you are done eating, you do not feel too heavy. Remember to eat only until you are 75% full. Snacking between meals is not supportive and should be avoided.

The Rhythm of Work

As we settle into adulthood, often our work schedule becomes fixed, as our employer demands a particular work hours. That work schedule, imposed upon us by outside forces, is often out of harmony with the rhythms of nature and this creates significant challenges. While self-employed individuals have greater control over their work schedules, employees will have to negotiate with their employers to establish a work rhythm that is harmonious.

When creating a harmonious work schedule, factors to consider are consistency, numbers of hours worked and adequate time off for lunch. In addition, workers who are forced to or choose to work overnight shifts will always develop an imbalance from being out of harmony with the rhythms of the sun and the moon.

Vata and the Healing Work Rhythm

If you have a vata nature or imbalance, it is very important that your work schedule be consistent. This helps you to stabilize the mobile quality of the vata dosha. Start times, break times and end times should be as consistent as possible.

When you break for lunch, it is important to take adequate time for the meal. While it may be tempting to work through lunch, this is very disharmonious and disturbs digestion. Thus, it is best to take at least one hour for lunch and, if possible, a little more time to allow for a walk in nature following the meal.

When an individual with a vata nature or imbalance is working, it is important to try and stay focused on only one task at a time. This is not always possible in a multi-tasking work environment but it will help to keep the vata dosha from moving further out of balance.

If you are required to work an overnight shift, by keeping all of your other rhythms steady and being consistent with your practices, you can minimize the harm that comes to you but you can not completely avoid an imbalance. If you have a significant imbalance and you are working an overnight shift – it's time to prepare for another job.

Pitta and the Healing Work Rhythm

Work is a serious event for those of you with a pitta nature. Many people with a pitta nature or imbalance are in leadership roles or are striving to be in one. The great challenge for you is to prevent yourself from becoming burned out by the process. To avoid burnout, it is important to keep to a regular work schedule with fixed start and end times and adequate time for a lunch break. People with a pitta nature or imbalance are the most likely to embrace long hours of work or working at home in the evenings. If this is true for you, remember this: If you burn out, you will be less productive over the long haul.

When you break for lunch, it is also important for you to take adequate time for the meal. While you may be motivated to work through lunch, this is very disharmonious and disturbs digestion. Thus, it is best to take at least one hour for lunch and, if possible, a little more time to allow for a walk in nature following the meal.

Discipline is needed in order to reign in the productive work spirit. It is helpful to schedule time for playful activities and to take those commitments as seriously as you do your work activities.

Kapha and the Healing Work Rhythm

When approaching work, a person with a kapha nature or imbalance may appear lazy to others. While this may be true at times, kapha's natural and healthy nature is to move about more slowly and with less intensity than other individuals. This affects how you approach your work as well. If you have a primary kapha nature, it is not likely that you are intensely focused on your goals. If this bothers your pitta boss, remind him or her that what you bring to your work is consistency, longevity and a steady work ethic. In fact, it is the person with a kapha nature that often achieves the most over the long haul, as burnout and distraction are less likely.

A steady work schedule is as helpful for a person with a kapha nature as it is for those with a vata or pitta nature. Variations in the work schedule, while being very disturbing to the nature of vata and pitta, are less disturbing for those with a kapha nature. In addition, a change in schedule or in responsibilities once in a while can be helpful for preventing stagnation.

When it comes to a lunch break, it is best to try and arrange a "brunch break", as 10:00 in the morning is the best time for your largest meal of the day. Taking a full hour for lunch allows for a relaxed meal that is well digested. It is best if you can work in enough time to allow for a quiet walk after the meal.

Recreation

As we grow into adult life and take on more and more responsibility, the role of play in our lives lessens. This is unfortunate, as play is very valuable to our well-being. Play helps to free the mind from becoming too serious and prevents the body from becoming too stagnant. Play itself is a form of rejuvenation. If you want to be as healthy as you can be, it is important to make the time for some healthy fun.

Recreation and the Vata Individual

Play for those of you with a vata nature comes a little easier than it might for those with a pitta or kapha nature as your light heart makes it easier to take things less seriously. While there are many forms of play and recreation, you are more likely to be drawn to creative forms of play such as art and drama. However, if your vata dosha is out of balance, these activities can be too light or etheric and can contribute to greater imbalance. At that time, grounding activities such as gardening, rock work or other activities that involve the earth is much better.

When you approach your recreation, be consistent. Include some recreation each day, even if it is just a half-hour of gardening when you get home from work. While a person with a balanced vata nature can engage in any playful form of recreation, if you have a vata imbalance, it is best to avoid activities that are too mobile and stimulating such as dance or aerobic classes.

Recreation and the Pitta Individual

For a person with a pitta nature and especially a person with a pitta imbalance, it is easy to turn play into a serious affair. While play is important, taking the seriousness out of the play is also important or it just becomes another form of work. While it is fun to compete, your pitta tendency is to focus on winning. Competitive play stokes your internal fire, building up the heat that leads to burnout. On the other hand, non-competitive play has a cooler and more stable nature and calms the fire.

It is your nature to turn anything that can be measured into a competition to improve your performance. This is true whether the competition is against an opponent or against yourself. If the results of a solitary activity can be measured, then you will strive to perform better and better. All of this is fine if there is no significant imbalance, but if there is an imbalance present, a non-competitive form of recreation will be healthier for you.

Examples of healthy non-competitive recreation can include going for a walk or hike, taking the boat out on the water or gardening. All of these are beneficial. Any activity that is less intellectual, less competitive, more body centered and performed in a relaxed manner will help to decrease the buildup of heat inside your body and mind.

Recreation and the Kapha Individual

For a person with a kapha nature or imbalance, an active form of play is very important and helpful for establishing balance. Your tendency is toward lethargy and this is made worse by sedentary work. Play offers the opportunity for you to get up and get moving.

Active forms of play increase the fire (energy) and the air (motivation). This is ideal for you, as it helps to keep body weight in balance, prevents the formation of mucus and stimulates the mind. Examples of healthy active forms of play include sports such as tennis, bicycling and aerobics classes. Competitive play is also beneficial as it may awaken some latent fire within.

Variations from the Daily Routine

As a general rule, it is best to avoid variations from your daily routine. A regular routine keeps vata dosha most in balance and helps to prevent pitta and kapha doshas from going out of balance. However, when it is not possible to keep the same routine every day, it may be possible to keep the same routine every week. In other words, if you can only play tennis on Tuesdays, make your schedule consistent so that your activity is every Tuesday at the same time. This is healthier than playing at different times each week. I call this "consistent variation" and this causes fewer imbalances than inconsistent variations. This same principle can be applied toward any aspect of the daily routine.

If you have a pitta or kapha nature, inconsistencies will have a less detrimental immediate impact. However, if they happen too often, they can cause your vata dosha to move out of balance which will then push your pitta or kapha doshas out of balance. This is more likely to occur with pitta dosha, which is not all that stable to begin with. When there is inconsistency, it is as if air is blowing on the fire. Often, this just makes the fire bigger. Kapha dosha is least disturbed by inconsistency and benefits from occasional spontaneity.

Daily Schedules

Below are sample daily schedules that bring balance to each of the three doshas. These schedules are ideals. You should not try to incorporate the full schedule into your life all at one time as this may be too overwhelming.

The Healthy Daily Schedule for Balancing Vata Dosha

Time of day	Activity
6:00 (sunrise)	Wake up, take a glass of warm water and start warming up some massage oil on the stove.
6:10	Sit to have a bowel movement
6:20	Self oil massage
6:30	Yoga and meditation practice
7:30	Breakfast
8:00	Take care of daily hygiene and get yourself dressed for the day (shower, floss, clean the eyes, neti)
8:30	Leave to work
9:00	Begin work
10:00	Light healthy snack
1:00	Lunch
4:00	Light healthy snack
5:00	End of work
7:00	Dinner
10:00	Bedtime

The Healthy Daily Schedule for Balancing Pitta Dosha

Time of day	Activity
5:30 (1/2 hour before sunrise)	Wake up, take a glass of warm water and start warming up some massage oil on the stove.
5:45	Sit to have a bowel movement
6:00	Self oil massage
6:15	Yoga and meditation practice
7:30	Breakfast
8:00	Take care of daily hygiene and get yourself dressed for the day (shower, floss, clean the eyes, neti)
8:30	Leave to work
9:00	Begin work
12:30	Lunch
5:00	End of work
6:00	Light dinner
10:00	Bedtime

The Healthy Daily Schedule for Balancing Kapha Dosha

Time of day	Activity
5:00 (1 hour before sunrise)	Wake up, take a glass of warm water and start warming up some massage oil on the stove.
5:15	Sit to have a bowel movement
5:30	Self oil massage with oil or powder
5:45	Yoga and meditation practice
7:00	Take a brisk morning walk
7:45	Take care of daily hygiene and get yourself dressed for the day (shower, floss, clean the eyes, neti)
8:30	Leave to work
9:00	Begin work
10:00	Brunch
5:00	End of work
6:00	Dinner
10:00	Bedtime

Personal Reflections

There is no doubt in my mind that creating a healthy daily routine is the most important of all of the concepts that Ayurveda teaches and that it is also the most difficult to implement in our lives. I have watched countless patients struggle with even the smallest changes and I have watched myself do the same. Our personal routine is a reflection of the very core of our nature, our consciousness. Changing our routines toward greater harmony means changing our values. When we are successful here we see the greatest transformation of our well-being.

Of course, there are endless distractions to making the transformation. In myself, my students and my patients, one great challenge I observe is that of having children. Those lovely little creatures wrap us around their fingers and soon our routine adapts to theirs. With school, carpools and making lunches, the morning gets taken up very quickly. Single moms have it the hardest of course, having to do it all alone and then if they have enough energy, they come home after work and help with homework. Somehow, meals are prepared and cleaning takes place. There is also the time spent playing games, going for walks, snuggling with a loved one and doing those things that families treasure. Between family and career, it is no wonder that it is difficult to establish a healthy routine.

But, what if you did not have a family? Would it be easier? From my observations of my patients and students who are single and without children, it is only marginally easier. The extra time gets eaten up by social activities and absorption into work.

So, what if you didn't have to work? Would it then become easier? Probably not. There are still social activities, community service and travel to distract you. After all, there are plans to make and life to manage.

What it really comes down to is priorities. When well-being is not a priority, everything else gets in the way. Once well-being becomes a priority, no matter what your life situation, you can make the transformation. The most important question is, just how important is harmony to you?

It took a long while for me to get into the routine of going to bed early and getting up early. Now I go to bed by 10:00 pm and sometimes earlier and get up between 5:30 and 6:00 am. That leaves me an hour for my practices in the morning before the rest of my family awakens. It's still not ideal; I'd like two hours but for now, that is where I am. Yoga, meditation and breathing practices fill up that hour. By doing my practices, the rest of my day is much more peaceful and I am less likely to get caught up in drama. My practices of morning neti and tongue scraping give me more energy. Ayurveda attributes this to the effect the practices have on my prana or life energy. Meanwhile, morning oil massage keeps my body strong and supple. It's a great day when I get up early.

It wasn't easy to make the transition. I used to stay up till about 11:00 or 11:30 and watch late night TV. I would watch the news, Leno or Letterman, The Daily Show or Stephen Colbert. Those last couple of hours before bed was "my time" after the kids went to bed and work was done. It was also a time that my wife and I would be together after a busy day. The shift began to happen for me when I had the opportunity to take some trips to a yoga ashram (Sivananda Yoga Center) to teach Ayurveda while living a yogic lifestyle –awakening at 5:30 to do morning meditation. Once I tasted the bliss of a healthy morning, I wanted to recreate that in my life. It took several years of wrestling with my habits before I was ready to consistently make the healthy choice of getting up and going to bed early and making time for my practices. I am by no means perfect. However, the result of my practices is that I experience much greater joy and all of the health benefits that come with it.

LESSON 15: THE MAN WHO CAME TO SEE LORD BUDDHA

In a small village in India there lived a man named Shambu who had attained a high status. He had plenty of money, a wife and children, a nice home and he was very successful in his work. Deep inside, however, he felt unfulfilled. One day, he heard that Lord Buddha was passing through his town. Having heard that this great teacher taught of fulfillment beyond material possessions, he decided to go and see the illumined holy man. As you might imagine, the line to see this great sage was very long, filled with people asking for his blessings. After many hours, his feet tired, his body hungry, he had his moment with the Brilliant One.

"Oh Lord Buddha" he began. " I have those things that most men seek. Yet still, I am not satisfied. I seek the enlightenment of which you speak. Please instruct me, and I will do all that you ask."

"Very well," Lord Buddha replied. " Give away all of your possessions. Leave your family and your work. Do you see that distant mountain? On the very top is a cave and outside of that cave is a tree. You are to live in that cave. You are to eat that which you can gather nearby and most of all, you are to live simply. Now, I will instruct you meditation and mantra. Listen closely."

The next day, Shambu took leave of his family and his possessions. Wearing only his most simple attire and carrying only water, he began his journey toward the mountain cave. For three weeks he hiked toward the mountaintop, stopping by streams to drink, eating the nuts and fruit he gathered and sleeping in soft beds he prepared from leaves. He arrived at the cave and it was exactly as the Great Rishi had described. Excited, he made it his home. Each day, he awoke and gathered his food from the surroundings. Each day he meditated under the Banyan Tree and repeated his mantras exactly as Lord Buddha had instructed him. As the days passed he felt no different. Still he was patient. Weeks passed and then months but still enlightenment eluded him. As the years passed, he faithfully stuck to his practices, at times wondering if perhaps he was doing something wrong.

One day, after nearly ten years had passed, a wandering forest dweller happened by and in passing mentioned that Lord Buddha would be again passing through their village. He decided that he would descend from the mountain and speak to the All-Knowing Sage. Of course, the line was again very long but after many hours, he appeared before the Brilliant One.

"Lord Buddha, you may not remember who I am," he began. "But many years ago, I came before you and asked what I needed to do in order to become enlightened. You instructed me to give up my possessions, leave my family, live simply in a cave up in the distant mountains and to meditate and chant." He repeated the instructions he had received in great detail and the Inspired Master nodded. "But Lord Buddha, I do not feel any more enlightened today than the day I first came to see you. Surely I am doing something wrong. Please, tell me what I am supposed to do."

Lord Buddha pondered his question in silence. After some time, he looked deep into Shambu's eyes. And, then he spoke. "I don't know." With that, he turned his back, and walked away.

Shambu stood still, frozen in his confusion. His lower jaw hung down, his eyes staring straight ahead. As the shock lessened, he began to wander aimlessly. His mind could not process what had just happened, Lord Buddha, the Brilliant One, the Enlightened Master did not know. He continued to wander but had nowhere to go. He no longer had a home, a family or a job.

After wandering for some time, Shambu stood still and recognizing that he needed shelter and food, he decided to walk back to the only home he had known for the past ten years. Along the way he lived off nuts and fruits and slept in beds of leaves. Upon arriving, he wondered for the first time what to do. After a moment of silence, he realized that it was late and he was tired and so he went to bed. When he awoke in the morning, he sat up and wondered what he would do with his day. In the silence, he realized that he was hungry and so he gathered from the offerings of a nearby field. After partaking of a delicious stew and then resting, he wondered again, what he would do next. He felt inspired to meditate and so he did, exactly as he always had and he repeated the mantra in the same way as he had always done. In that moment, under the Banyan tree, Shambu knew great peace. He felt satisfied and tears of joy rolled down his face. Then, he began to laugh and laugh and laugh and he could not stop. Soon the trees, the wind, the water and the sun were all laughing with him and their laughter became harmony and their voice was One.

REFERENCES AND RESOURCES

Classical Ayurvedic Textbooks

Ashtang Hrdayam: Translated by Prof. K.R. Srikantha Murthy, ©1994, Krishnadas Academy, Varanasi, India.

Ashtang Samgraha: Translated by Prof. K.R. Srikantha Murthy, ©1995, Chaukhambha Orientalia, Varanasi, India.

Caraka Samhita: Translated by R.K. Sharma and Bhagwan Dash, ©1992, Chaukhambha Sanskrit Series Office, Varanasi, India.

Madhava Nidanam: Translated by K.R.L. Gupta, ©1997, Sri Satguru Publications, a division of Indian Books Centre, New Delhi, India.

Sarangadhara Samhita: Translated by Prof. K.R. Srikantha Murthy, ©1995, Chaukhambha Orientalis, Varanasi, India.

Sushruta Samhita: Translated by K.L. Bhishagratna, ©1991, Chaukhambha Sanskrit Series Office, Varanasi, India.

Dravya Guna Vijnanam

Supplemental Ayurvedic Resources

American Institute of Vedic Studies: Correspondence Text, Dr. David Frawley

Principles of Ayurvedic Medicine: Textbook of the California College of Ayurveda: Dr. Marc Halpern

Plant, Essential Oils and Aroma Therapy References

USDA Natural Resource Conservation Service: http://plants.usda.gov

Esoteric Oils Database: "http://www.essentialoils.co.za/essential-oils"

Complete Book of Essential Oils: Valerie Ann Worwood, ©1991, New World Library, San Rafael, California

Ayurveda and Aromatherapy: Drs. Light and Bryan Miller, ©1995, Lotus Press, Wisconsin

Indigenous Drugs of India: 2nd edition, 1896, Kanny Lal Dey, Calcutta/Great Britain

Plants for a Future: "http://www.pfaf.org/database/plants.php "http://www.pfaf.org/database/plants.php

Environmental Protection Agency: "http://www.epa.gov/"

HerbalPedia Herbal Database A-Z: "http://www.herbalmedicine/"

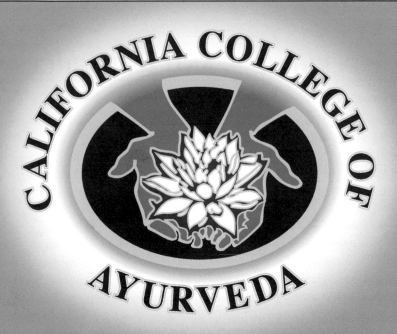

CALIFORNIA COLLEGE OF AYURVEDA